World Vision

Violence Against Women:

From Silence to ***Empowerment***

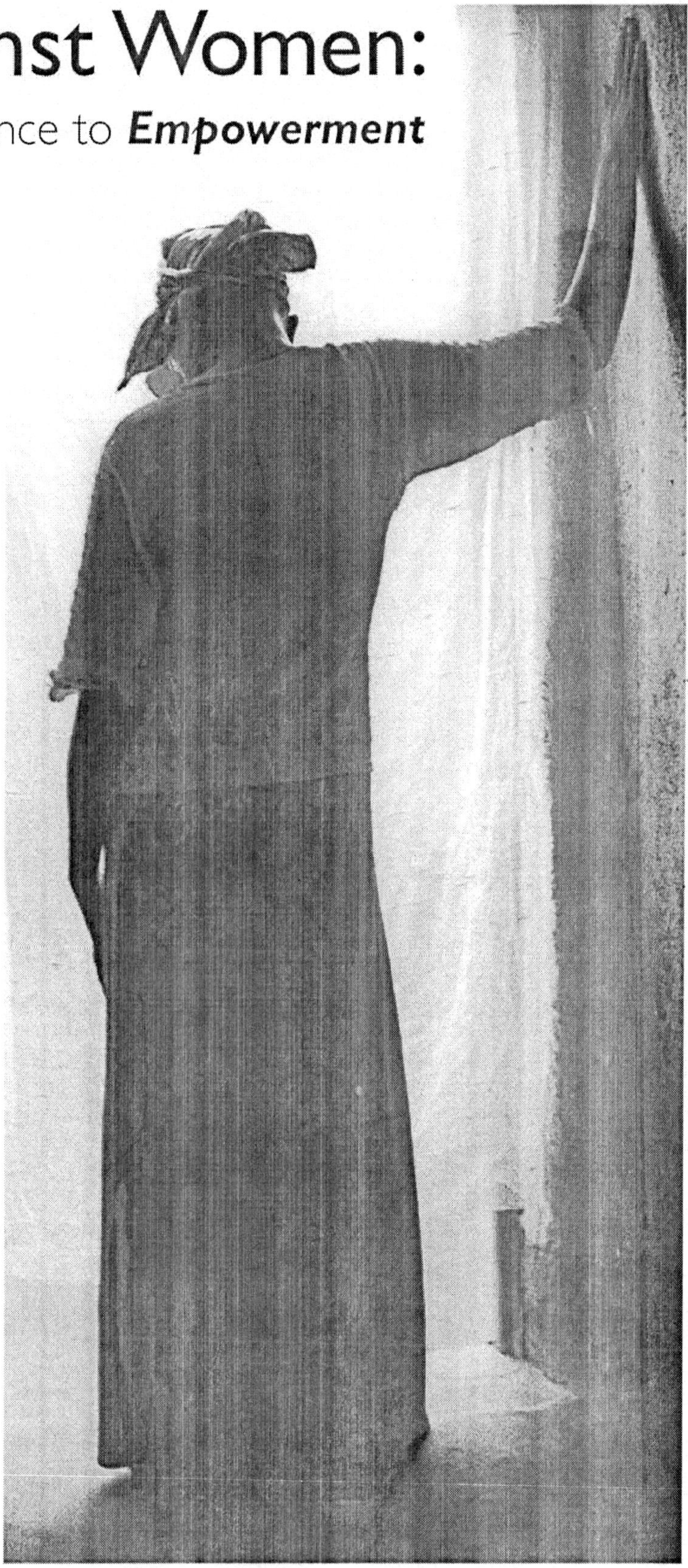

Edited by
Don Brandt

Foreword by
Fatuma Hashi

Violence Against Women

From Silence to Empowerment

Edited by Don Brandt

Foreword by Fatuma Hashi

World Vision

Printed in USA

Published by World Vision International, 800 West Chestnut Avenue, Monrovia, California 91016-3198, U.S.A.

ISBN 1-887983-54-6

Editor in chief: Edna Valdez. Senior Editor: Rebecca Russell. Copyeditor: Heather Elliott Typesetting: Richard Sears. Cover design: Judy Walker. Cover photo: Alison Preston

Printed on recycled paper.

Contributors

Sara Austin (*Commercial sexual exploitation of children: How extra-territorial legislation can help*) is Child Rights Policy Analyst at World Vision Canada. She works on issues related to children and youth participation in their own development, impact of HIV/AIDS on girls, and general concerns of the girl child. Sara has a keen interest in curbing gender-based violence through creating enabling environments where boys and girls can become agents of change.

Alejandro Cartes co-authored (*Domestic violence: Aggression against women in Chile*) with Paula Saez. Like Paula, Alejandro works with World Vision Chile as a journalist. He has an abiding interest in poverty, justice and violence, both in families and communities. Alejandro believes that it's primarily through families that new and more peaceful social relationships are formed and sustained.

Heather Elliott (*Introduction*) has worked with World Vision Australia (WVA) in many capacities. For the past eight years she served with WVA's Advocacy Network. Heather is active in issues of peace and conflict, including the campaign to ban landmines. She edited several reports, including *Children and Peacebuilding* and this volume.

Brenda Fitzpatrick (*Rape as genocide: Lessons from the Balkans and Rwanda in the 1990s*) worked and travelled in many areas of conflict. These experiences provided her with first-hand materials to advocate, write and speak on a wide range of topics dealing with human rights and development. Brenda's work experience includes senior management positions at the World Council of Churches, World Vision Australia and, currently, World Association of Girl Guide and Girl Scouts.

Ruth Kahurananga (*Finding a way forward: Gender-based violence in Tanzania*) was manager of World Vision Tanzania's Advocacy Unit while serving as the gender and development (GAD) focal person. In these positions, Ruth was able to lead team research efforts on topics related to gender-based violence and the promotion of child rights. Ruth now works with World Vision International as Child Rights Policy Officer, based in New York.

Frieda Kana (*Family and sexual violence in Papua New Guinea*) is Communications and Information Technology Manager at World Vision Papua New Guinea. Frieda experienced first hand the all-pervasive repression of women in Papuan culture. She remains hopeful, seeing improvements that include universal education regardless of sex and the emergence of women's rights activities and organisations.

Monalisa Kileo co-authored (*Finding a way forword: Gender-based violence in Tanzania*) with Ruth Kahurananga. Trained as a journalist, Monalisa's works with World Vision Tanzania as Correspondence Analyst. Her interest in gender and violence against women dates to her college years and her BA thesis on increased divorce in Tanzania.

Sylvia Mpaayei (*Violence against women in Europe*) serves on the staff of World Vision United Kingdom as contact person on gender issues and as Programme Development Officer. A native of Kenya, Sylvia's interest in gender began when she worked with groups of women who faced conflict and brutality in Sudan. She believes that in too many societies a "culture of silence" condones violence against women. Sylvia feels that one role of development organisations is to support women facing violence and empower them to make wise decisions about their own well-being.

Paula Sáez (*Domestic violence: Aggression against women in Chile*) is a trained journalist on the staff of World Vision Chile. Paula believes that all of us should be advocates for victims of domestic violence, re-

gardless of whom the abused may be. Her desire is to put faces on violence, and by so doing, achieve greater consciousness about the tragedy of domestic violence.

Dr Sekai Shand (*The links between HIV/AIDS and violence: Towards a dialogue with men*) is manager of the Advocacy, Media and Public Relations Department at World Vision Australia. Sekai, born in Zimbabwe, completed her education in Britain and Australia. Her passion for poverty and development concerns undergirds her professional work and writing. That same fervour is strikingly found in Sekai's fictional stories, including *Songs to an African Sunset*.

Contents

Foreword

Violence against women is a crime against humanity. It is first and foremost a violation of human rights. Physical, sexual and psychological abuses are an affront to the dignity and intrinsic worth of every individual. Rape, trafficking of women and girls, early and forced marriage and female genital mutilation are human rights abuses that occur too frequently, in too many communities. And no society, not even in "enlightened" Western Europe, is exempt from the scourge of domestic violence, robbing a woman of the sanctity and security of her home.

Violence against women is also a barrier to development. World Vision and other development agencies have long recognised that only with the active participation of women can development be sustainable. Development programs that ignore repression and subjugation of women are doomed to failure. Women are the primary care givers of children. Meeting the basic needs of children extends to economic production, whether growing crops, working as petty traders or serving as corporate executives.

As a human rights and development desecration, indeed a grave humanitarian concern, violence against women demands responses at all levels: from individual and family through community, national and international levels. Nothing short of personal and cultural behavioural transformations are called for. The battle has been joined and there has been change – despite the continuation of despicable acts, such as commercial sexual exploitation, "honour killing" and rape as an act of war. Perhaps the question to ask is: "How will each of us be engaged with this issue in our home, work, and civic lives?"

Endorsement of the Convention on the Elimination of All Forms of Discrimination against Women (CEDAW) is a testimony to the importance World Vision places on combating gender discrimination as a blight on humankind.

This book is not intended as an academic exercise alone. It serves as a communiqué against forms of violence that are perpetuated against too many human beings. The authors want to convey the sheer extent to which fundamental human rights of women are being violated; to unpack the distorted personal and societal attitudes that this ultimately reflects; and to remind us that it need not be this way.

Fatuma Hashi
Gender and Development Director
World Vision International

Introduction

So God created humankind in his image...
male and female he created them.

– *Genesis 1:27*

Now the earth was corrupt in God's sight,
and the earth was filled with violence...
and it grieved [God] to his heart.

– *Genesis 6:11, 6*

Everyone has the right to life, liberty
and security of person.

–*Article 3, Universal Declaration of Human Rights, 1948*

Violence against Women: From Silence to Empowerment brings together some perspectives from around the world on the pressing issue of violence against women and girls. The authors show that gender-based violence has diverse manifestations and that the scale of the problem is enormous, in both its severity and spread. Indeed, the stories and perspectives from diverse parts of the world represented in this book have numerous tragic elements in common.

While not claiming to be comprehensive in its analysis, *Violence against Women: From Silence to Empowerment* offers valuable insights both into the far-reaching impacts of gender-based violence on human development and into measures that offer hope of effectively reducing this violence and its impacts. What becomes clear is how often the route out of violence and fear is dependent on chance and the work of local community organisations. Our case studies show that women have few obvious places to turn when they are at risk and suffering abuse. In most countries provision for the victims of domestic violence are inadequate and poorly advertised. Where limited exceptions occur (such as Chile) they stand out as beacons for other countries to follow.

The World Health Organisation reported in October 2002[1] that violence is now the leading cause of death among people aged 15 to 44. More than 1.6 million people are killed by violence each year; for every person killed by violence, as many as 40 people are left with serious injuries as a result of physical attacks. Yet violence, particularly against women, rarely features in global policy commitments or the pronouncements of the G8. Eradicating domestic violence is not a Millennium Development Goal and it is disturbingly absent from most Poverty Reduction Strategy Papers.

The lack of attention given to violence against women in the policy debate is reflected in most countries by a failure of government action. This report calls for renewed scrutiny of the problem of violence against women as an issue that must not be ignored by those who work in and for development. Action is urgently needed to build on the positive lessons highlighted in these case studies. In particular there is a need to build the capacity of local government and civil society organisations to address the problem of violence and to raise the awareness among women of their rights.

World Vision's experience is that the scale and pervasiveness of violence against women, during war and peace, both within and outside the home, means that humanitarian organisations encounter forms of physical and sexual abuse in nearly all childcare, development and relief program contexts. If an organisation is serious about transformational development of human lives, it cannot ignore brutality against women and girls.

It is clear that violence against women by men is widespread with serious, even deadly, impacts. The fact is that men are the most common perpetrators of violence and of sexual abuse against women and girls. Men almost always have superior physical force, with the obvious result that their violence can threaten or inflict acute, even life-threatening, physical harm.

In this book, authors tell of hospital admissions, rapes and murders resulting from domestic violence; of girls sold into sexual slavery; of women suffering severe pain, sickness and eventual death as a result of infection with HIV by their husbands. Furthermore, in far more families and societies, women are *dependent* on men – including violent men – for their physical survival. The economic and social power over women that societies allows men to claim means that many women are trapped in situations of violence, without real alternatives. This creates situations that, like that of children abused by their parents or primary caregivers, are utterly horrific. As one author in this book notes, "the psychological impact of domestic violence has been found to have parallels with the impact of torture and imprisonment of hostages."

In armed conflict, when human potential for evil acts tends to have freer reign than usual, women are not the only victims of violence and inhumanity; civilians in general suffer gross violations of the international rules of war. But women are victims in particular ways. The International Committee of the Red Cross has in recent years documented the impact of armed conflict on women, and called for recognition of the specific problems women face in conflict, including mutilation, sexual violence, the loss of husbands and sons, and inadequate protection.[2]

Sexual violence is in a special sense an invasion of a woman's person, of sexual organs that are intended both to provide intimacy and delight between loved ones, and to create and nurture new human life.

Impacts on development

The impacts of gender-based violence on the development process are reason enough for humanitarian organisations to be concerned about the issue.

Where women are violently abused, whole families are held back from fulfilling their potential spiritually, socially or economically. Women who are physically injured or traumatised have less energy to study, educate or nourish their children, carry out income-generating activities, farming, carrying water or other household and community tasks. Violence ultimately affects the contribution of women to the development of a nation.

Where violence against women occurs on a broad scale, relationships in the community can be marked by gender division, bitterness and a culture of silence or apathy, all of which work against community-based development.

Sexual violence against girls and women often leads to the victims withdrawing from (or being shunned by) their family or community, or even becoming infected with HIV, with all the implications that AIDS has for development.

...on children

World Vision and other child-focused organisations are also concerned with this issue because of our commitment to a world that is safe for children.

Children are directly and profoundly impacted by violence against women. As some of the chapters in this book reveal, both female and male children clearly learn violence and gender discrimination in childhood, and *reproduce* violent relationships in their homes when they grow up; for some, tragically, abuse is a normal way of relating in the family. Sexual violence also dramatically affects children's ability to form healthy, loving relationships as adults. No child – male or female – should have to experience at close hand, particularly within the closest human bond known to them (the family), the invasion of violence. Whether they suffer, witness, overhear or find themselves mediating, children are profoundly affected by acts of violence in their own homes. More than one chapter makes the point that violence against women is violence against families.

Rape that results in pregnancy represents violence against the bond between a mother and her children. Indeed, children born of the rapes committed in Rwanda and the Balkans are known as "unwanted" and in many cases even killed by those who give birth to them.

...on women themselves

But it is not only because of children that humanitarian organisations are concerned about violence against women. They are troubled because of their commitment to the marginalised and vulnerable. As noted in World Vision's Faces of Violence report,[3]

women as a group are often among the most marginalised.

The authors insist that women equally with men are precious in God's sight, and possess the same innate dignity and human rights. Gender-based violence is specifically and comprehensively proscribed in the *Declaration against Violence against Women*,[4] adopted by the UN General Assembly in 1993, and the *Platform for Action from the UN Fourth World Conference on Women*[5] in 1995. Both of these documents define gender-based violence as a violation of human rights, and also as a form of discrimination that prevents women from participating fully in society and fulfilling their potential as human beings.

Violence against women is not specifically proscribed in the *Convention on the Elimination of All Forms of Discrimination Against Women* (CEDAW), which has been ratified by 170 countries[6], however the CEDAW States Parties commit themselves to:

> take in all fields, in particular in the political, social, economic and cultural fields, all appropriate measures, including legislation, to ensure the full development and advancement of women, for the purpose of guaranteeing them the exercise and enjoyment of human rights and fundamental freedoms on a basis of equality with men (Article 3);
>
> take all appropriate measures... to modify the social and cultural patterns of conduct of men and women, with a view to achieving the elimination of prejudices and customary and all other practices which are based on the idea of the inferiority or the superiority of either of the sexes or on stereotyped roles for men and women (Article 5);
>
> take all appropriate measures, including legislation, to suppress all forms of traffic in women and exploitation of prostitution of women (Article 6);
>
> take all appropriate measures to eliminate discrimination against women in all matters relating to marriage and family relations (Article 16).

Causes

There are different theories as to the causes of violence against women, and the authors touch on numerous of these: violence may be motivated by an individual's desire to exert power (Austin), to "intimidate, punish or humiliate" the woman or girl (Kahurananga & Kileo), or to demonstrate one's masculinity (Shand, Kana);

The authors from Chile (Sáez & Cartes) share the profound observation of one social scientist that "violence has its origins in the denial of the other person's truth in order to obtain obedience and subjection." Adultery and jealousy are other reasons given for wife battery.

In some cases there are unmistakable cultural and societal roots that cause violence against women to be accepted and even encouraged. Many women themselves accept it as something they must endure; a notable reluctance of many law enforcers to intervene and prosecute domestic or sexual violence indicates they tend to agree. Patriarchal ideology and power and control exercised by men as a group over women, are also mentioned as key factors. Moreover, as noted in World Vision's *Faces of Violence* report, in a context where many acts of violence are committed by the state against citizens, and where whole societies have become accustomed to armed violence, some of the barriers to violence no longer exist.

It is clear that poverty is a major contributor, and this is where the issue becomes critically relevant for humanitarian organisations. Poverty *itself* is violence. But, as highlighted by the *Faces of Violence* report, strong links can be made between poverty and deep social inequities, and violence. The enormous stresses facing families in poverty drive some people to lash out violently; as one author puts it: "Poverty pushes people past the limits of their patience."

Poverty also drives people to treat their own daughters as commodities to be sold, whether that be to a well-off older man, in exchange for a bride price, or to a recruiter of the sex trade (perhaps in the belief that they will supply a decent form of employment). At least three of the authors point to changes

associated with modernisation as a significant factor that contributes to violence against women. These include rural–urban dislocation and separation of families, which are key factors in the HIV infection of married women by their husbands. Poverty that forces parents to remove their daughters from school at an early age also increases the chances that she will not be armed with knowledge sufficient to protect herself from either abusive relationships or that disease.

Also linked are physiological factors. It is well known that the consumption of alcohol in many cases fans the flames of violence. What of the effects of hunger or malnourishment on the human mind and emotions? One anthropological study[7] linked malnourishment contributing to low blood-sugar levels with one community's endemic aggression and violence. If, as is now generally believed, chemical and electrical impulses in the brain exert influence over one's emotional and physiological impulses, what happens to children who are deprived of nutrition or affection at critical junctures of their development?

Are men always to blame? For the acts of violence they carry out, there can be no other answer but "yes" – otherwise we are denying human responsibility for one's own actions. There is no doubt that strained relationships, exhaustion and stress caused by overwork, injustice or chronic poverty can shorten one's fuse. But there is a huge distinction between getting angry and inflicting violence that causes physical injury or death.

Even in courts of law, blaming the victim of violence is common. In my own country, Australia, a woman brutally murdered by her ex-partner was said to have "provoked" the crime. To the horror of the woman's family, the killer received a short prison sentence.[8] Yet a woman charged with the murder of her husband after suffering decades of abuse and cruelty at his hands, was not able to claim provocation to the satisfaction of the court, and received a long prison sentence.[9]

Solutions

Laws criminalising violence against women are critical, as all the authors note. When countries publicly acknowledge the problem, such as by introducing legislation or welfare interventions in response to domestic violence or sexual, the issue moves from the private to the public sphere. Victims begin to have a small hope of vindication and perpetrators begin to tremble. Societies that take such steps may be shocked at the extent of these problems in their midst that were previously hidden now comes to light.

Laws alone are not enough. Clearly, the number of cases reported is still only the tip of the iceberg, and the number of convictions pitifully low. The challenge is to disseminate laws against abuse in a manner that is understandable, particularly to people who are not educated or live in remote areas.

Most of the authors agree that social education and awareness programs, and the creation of new norms, also continue to be a major need, particularly where culture or traditional practices (such as female genital mutilation) are involved. One author notes that positive traditional beliefs can be harnessed to empower and protect women. Community attitudes can be changed through education about the adverse health, psychological and socio-economic effects of violence.

Violence against women: a men's issue

As several of the authors highlight, men and boys are critical to solving the problem of gender-based violence. Yet they may have few resources available to help them should they want to overcome the problem in themselves or in their communities. Many may not have awareness of or access to non-violent models or alternatives, or may have difficulty in articulating their thoughts and feelings. Sadly, many have not been targeted by NGOs purporting to address the problem of violence against women.

The importance of empowering boys and girls, men and women, "in such a way that the rights of all people are respected and nurtured" (Austin) is underlined. Several authors note the need for alternative masculine identities, ones that do not "require" a man to beat his wife in order to prove his virility or strength. Education, peer groups or the media can provide credible non-violent role models or approaches.

The church is noted by many of the authors as having a special role, both in providing space where people's concerns on issues such as violence could be expressed, and families could be supported in dealing with the problem, and in providing an authoritative moral basis for promoting abstinence and monogamous sexual relations as a critical element of reducing the transmission of HIV/AIDS. Yet, several authors point out, the church also needs to examine its own complicity in the disempowerment of women.

Development agencies such as World Vision have opportunities to identify and address, on many different levels, issues of violence against women. Several of the authors make specific recommendations for programming and advocacy to this end.

Barriers

Barriers to recognising and solving gender-based violence are identified, ranging from inadequate compilation of data from a range of welfare and law enforcement agencies, and lack of data on sexual exploitation that is disaggregated by gender and age; female poverty and lack of participation in decision-making, education and employment; women's lack of power to negotiate safe sex, even if they know what it is; to unclear processes and policies at government level. The failure of government agencies to respond to the needs of women is an acute problem and the need for an ethos of service provision that includes the rights of women is clear.

Almost all the chapters in this book refer to a "culture of silence" that surrounds violence against women. Many women are reluctant to report domestic violence or rape. In Chile it is reported that women wait on average seven years from when the problem starts until they file a complaint. The silence is often due to women's shame in letting others know about violence, fear of retribution or dependence, whether emotional, social or economic, on their abusers. Others do not know where they can turn for help.

World Vision is conscious that women are often let down by those who should be willing and able to help – law enforcement agencies, local authorities and also civil society. In developing countries, however, services for women are also in turn victims, neglected by bilateral donors or international financial institutions.

Poverty Reduction Strategies increasingly focus on a few development goals that neither donors nor lenders should overlook the crucial needs of women and the role that they play in overcoming poverty. World Vision would suggest that taking a more rights-based approach to their work would help agencies that work with governments in the social policy sphere (such as the World Bank) to better identify and address problems such as violence against women, although sadly the Bank has been reluctant to adopt such an approach.

Silence protects those who abuse women. For this reason – for these crimes to be seen for what they are – the silence must be broken. World Vision publishes this report to further this end.

Violence against women is a human rights violation and an affront to the image of God. Not only women, but also men, need liberation from violence – from patterns of thinking and action that devalue and destroy human life rather than nurture it, that undermine one's own ability to protect the weak, and that send ripples across society and into future generations. If humanity can be viewed as a fabric that is knitted together, then one person inflicting or suffering violence, however subtle, stains and unravels that fabric. May this book challenge us all to identify and deal with the traces of violence in ourselves, our communities and our world.

The chapters

Paula Sáez and Alejandro Cartes examine the serious concern of *Domestic violence: Aggression against women in Chile*. Dimensions of the problem are presented in statistical data (one recent study found that over 50% of women in Chile have experienced violent situations in their relationships with their partners) and one woman's personal story. While violence against women is clearly endemic – the authors suggest it is enshrined in the national motto – the tireless efforts of civil society organisations including the church have yielded fruit. Chile has in-

troduced important initiatives such as the Law on Domestic Violence, and the establishment of a National Service for Women. The issue is now clearly in the public sphere, and recognised for the crime that it is, where once it was hidden in families.

Nevertheless, limitations with the implementation of the Law have meant a failure to protect victims and witnesses, while social inequity and poverty render many abused women dependent on their abusers and unwilling or unable to bring them to justice. Awareness-raising campaigns continue to be critical in building new social norms. This chapter shows how World Vision Chile is addressing the issue proactively and comprehensively, through programs focusing on individuals and family relationships, economic development to address poverty, and advocacy and awareness-raising to build a new "culture" of peace and respect.

Sekai Nzenza Shand, in *The links between HIV/AIDS and violence: Towards a dialogue with men,* shows how the disempowerment of women, at family, village and national levels, increases their vulnerability to both sexual violence and the added violence of HIV infection. Many Southern African women, particularly in rural areas, lack both knowledge of and control over their sexuality: this means less power in a relationship to negotiate the use of condoms to protect their own health. Traditional practices and beliefs are examined, including widespread double standards for men and women where sexual behaviour is concerned. This chapter argues that men have a critical role in tackling the AIDS epidemic, but that opportunities to include them, and to nurture alternative masculine identities, have too often been missed. It concludes with recommendations for programming and advocacy to meet these urgent challenges.

Sara Austin addresses the violence of child sexual exploitation, which particularly impacts girls and inflicts physical, emotional and psychological trauma on its victims. Countless girls are held virtually as prisoners in the sex trade – often to repay family debts, unaware of who might help them escape to a different reality. *Commercial sexual exploitation of children: How extra-territorial legislation can help* focuses on child sex tourism and trafficking, and the critical importance of extra-territorial legislation in tackling these cross-border crimes. The strengths and weaknesses of legal measures enacted by five tourist-sending countries are assessed. There have been very few prosecutions to date. This chapter calls for "an international social and political climate where the commercial sexual exploitation of children will no longer be tolerated, and where there is no impunity for offenders." Noting that these problems exist within an international social context that tolerates and perpetuates gender-based violence, it argues that strategies must address the imbalance of power between men and women, and between adults and children.

Ruth Kahurananga and Monalisa Kileo, in their chapter *Finding a way forward: Gender-based violence in Tanzania,* present three different types of gender-based violence that are prevalent in Tanzania: domestic violence extends beyond physical violence to psychological (threats, intimidation, isolating a woman from her friends and family, and economic control); various forms of female genital mutilation; and the accusation and killing of elderly women for "witchcraft." They discuss the devastating impacts and various root causes (economic, cultural and otherwise) of these forms of violence; efforts that have been made by government and civil society in Tanzania to eradicate them; and some suggestions to meet the challenges that remain.

Brenda Fitzpatrick's chapter, *Rape as genocide: Lessons from the Balkans and Rwanda in the 1990s,* focuses on the horrific (both in scale and nature) sexual abuses of women in those conflicts. It is clear that thousands of women fell victim to this humiliation, pain and terror. This chapter traces efforts to ensure that rape is acknowledged as being useable not only as a weapon of war, but also a tool of genocide, carried out with "the specific intent to destroy, in whole or in part, a particular group." Much hinges on whether the rapes were planned and systematic, rather than opportunistic. Certainly, some perpetrators considered raping a greater violence than killing their victims, allowing them instead to "die of sadness"; some sought to impregnate their victims

so that they would bear children of the perpetrator's ethnicity. Obstacles to enforcing and prosecuting genocidal rape include an attitude that acts of sexual violence against women are "lesser crimes," and issues of state sovereignty.

Sylvia Mpaayei reports high levels of *Violence against women in Europe* – lest the reader assume that gender-based violence is a problem of developing countries. While some types of violence, such as trafficking in women, appear to be more prevalent in Eastern European countries, domestic violence is alarmingly common in the United Kingdom. This chapter presents data on Europeans' attitudes to domestic violence against women, its causes and how they believe it should be tackled. Discussed are recent initiatives in the European Community and the UK, including by the church, to tackle and prevent violence against women including trafficking. In Europe, as elsewhere, women do not always report the crimes committed against them. A woman's capacity or willingness to take steps to protect herself from violence depends on her awareness of alternatives and support services, as well as on levels of support from children and other relatives, and her economic situation.

Frieda Kana presents *Family and sexual violence in Papua New Guinea* as a human rights concern that has reached critical proportions. She presents data and stories from personal experience that indicates both the pervasiveness of domestic violence and its apparent acceptance by society. An increase in sexual violence, including rape, is also highlighted. Tragically, it has taken cases of extreme brutality to raise public awareness of the seriousness of these problems. Exploring both the perceived and the underlying causes (that include cultural beliefs and gender identities, and stress caused by rapid socio-economic change) of such violence, this chapter reports on legislative and civil society efforts that have helped bring these issues into the open.

References

[1] World Health Organization, *World Report on Violence and Health*, Geneva, October 2002, http://www.who.int/violence_injury_prevention/main.cfm/p=0000000117

[2] International Committee of the Red Cross, Women facing War, ICRC, Geneva, 2001. The report can be read on-line at http://www.icrc.org/Web/eng/siteeng0.nsf/iwpList2/Focus:Women_and_War. At the launch of this report, President of the ICRC, Jakob Kellenberger, made a declaration calling for greater recognition of the specific needs and vulnerabilities of women in wartime.

[3] World Vision, *Faces of Violence in Latin America and the Caribbean* (available in Spanish and English), World Vision International, Regional Office for Latin America and the Caribbean, San José, Costa Rica, 2002. See also Don Brandt, Homes of Fear: The Curse of Family Violence, Working Paper No. 6, World Vision International, Monrovia, CA, May 2002.

[4] http://www.unhchr.ch/huridocda/huridoca.nsf/(Symbol)/A.RES.48.104.En?Opendocument

[5] http://www.un.org/womenwatch/daw/beijing/platform/violence.htm

[6] As at 9 December 2002 http://www.unhchr.ch/html/menu3/b/e1cedaw.htm

[7] R. Bolton's study of the Qolla, an Aymará-speaking group in the South American Andes, referenced in R. M. Keesing, *Cultural Anthropology: A Contemporary Perspective*, CBS College Publishing, New York, 1981, pp. 95–96.

[8] In August 1987, Vicki Cleary, a kindergarten teacher in Melbourne was stabbed to death by her ex-boyfriend in a car park. Her killer argued that she had provoked him and received only three and a half years' imprisonment for manslaughter. The victim's brother wrote that the judge "granted a defence of provocation because '...there were acts and circumstances existing for some time before-

hand which, in culmination...produced a loss of self-control because of the trigger comment that occurred that day by the deceased lady.' The 'trigger comment' was an exclamation allegedly uttered by my sister upon being confronted at...her car. The circumstances were her refusal to return to a violent relationship. An earlier appearance at the kindergarten by the aggressive [killer] was described by the judge as: 'part of a realistic situation (where) one person is intense about seeing the other'." 'The legal lie that men kill for love', *The Age*, Melbourne, 19 August 1998. http://www.philcleary.com.au/politics_murder_legal_lie.htm

9 In October 1996, Heather Osland (R v Osland [1998] 2 VR 636) was found guilty of murdering her husband, and sentenced to 14 years' imprisonment. "At her trial, she pleaded both self-defence and provocation, on the basis that she was fearful for her life, due to a long-standing history of violence against both her and her son by her husband. Her conviction and sentence were unsuccessfully appealed [to two Courts]. Critics of these decisions have argued that the law of self-defence and provocation is gender biased, and is incapable of taking into account the context of violence in which such killings occur." Defences to Homicide: Issues paper, Victorian Law Reform Commission, Melbourne, 2002, p. 17, s. 1.19. http://www.lawreform.vic.gov.au/CA256902000FE154/Lookup/Homicide/$file/Issues_Paper.pdf

Vicki Cleary's brother, commenting on the Osland case, said: "One must wonder what Heather Osland, sentenced to 15 years for the murder of her pathologically violent husband, would make of suggestions that our courts are free of notions of male honour or gender bias. Despite Osland's son wielding the piece of pipe that killed her husband, he was freed. And although Justice Kirby relied heavily on the "sanctity of human life" when rejecting Osland's appeal...some have asked whether flawed cultural assumptions and the sanctity of man's place in the home weren't the real sub-text."

Domestic violence: Aggression against women in Chile

Paula Sáez and Alejandro Cartes

Introduction

> "They beat you so much, so much, that they make you believe you are insignificant; you end up believing it." – *Aída Moreno*

Since she was six years old, Aída Moreno[1] has known beatings, forced labour and discrimination as a way of life. The sadness in her eyes reflects a life marked by physical and psychological abuse.

Aída and her siblings were punished violently by her stepmother, who had been authorised by Aída's father to beat them; his belief was that "as long as their eyes and mouths aren't hurt, the rest doesn't matter."

Originally from Chanco, a town in Maule province deep in the countryside, Aída arrived in Santiago, the capital city when she was only 14 years of age. At 15, she was raped by the man who would later become her husband. The violence she experienced during her childhood was repeated in adult life. The harsh situation in which she lived, however, did not dampen her interest in helping others. Ultimately, Aída was able to recognise herself as a person loved by God, to understand her situation and begin the struggle to find herself as a woman. (More of Aída's story appears later in this paper.)

Aída is not alone. In the Santiago region, one out of every three women has been the object of physical and/or sexual violence. In addition, psychological violence is known by one in every 10 women.[2]

Por la Razón o la Fuerza – "Through Reason or Force" – is the national slogan of Chile. It also encapsulates how a large number of Chilean men think and act, using violence as a way of imposing "respect" in their homes.

The couple: one aggressor, the other injured

Domestic violence, of which women are the primary victims, is a cause for serious concern in Chilean society. In 1992, with support from the Pan-American Health Organization (PAHO), a study on *The Prevalence of Family Violence in Chile*[3] reported the shocking reality of domestic abuse: in 25% of households, the woman was beaten by her spouse; in 30% of these cases, she was psychologically abused as well.

A later study on the prevalence of domestic violence, completed in 2001, indicated that 50.35% of Chilean women have experienced violent situations in their relationships with their partners. Of these, over 32% suffered psychological violence and 67.5% experienced physical abuse. The report shows that domestic violence occurs in all strata of society: among 38% of women from the upper and upper–middle income group, 44.8% of middle class women, and 59.4% of women in the low-income sector.[4]

A recent study by the National Service for Women (SERNAM) highlights that:

- in the Santiago Metropolitan Region alone, the problem affects 50.3% women between the ages of 15 and 49, and more than 70% of children.
- nationally, one in every two married or separated women has suffered – at least once – violence from her partner. Meanwhile, three out of four children have suffered some kind of violence at the hands of their parents.
- women with higher educational levels are less likely to suffer violence at the hands of their partners. The prevalence of physical violence amongst women who have not completed their primary or high school education stands at 40%; in contrast, the rate for those who have completed high school is 29.1%, while for women who have completed their university studies it stands at 28.5%.

Table 1: Data on domestic violence in Chile

Year	Source	Findings
1992	Larraín (supported by PAHO)	• women beaten by spouse in 25% of households • psychological abuse in 30% of these cases
2001	Public Policy Analysis Centre (Chile)	• 50.35% of women had experienced violence in relationships with partners • 34% of these physical violence • 16.3% psychological violence • highest rates of violence in low-income sector • in the Metropolitan Region alone, domestic violence affects 50.3% women aged 15–49, and more than 70% of children • nationally, one in every two married or separated women has suffered violence from her partner, and three out of four children have suffered violence at the hands of their parents • prevalence of violence lowers as women's education levels increase: • 40% among women who have not completed primary or high school • 29.1% for women who have completed high school • 28.5% for women who have completed university studies
2002	Citizen Security Division, Ministry of the Interior	• 32,515 reported cases in second trimester of 2002 – 12.3% more than second trimester 2001

- in relationships where there is violence, there is an increasing tendency for threats to be made at gunpoint: some 20% of the women who have faced serious physical violence at home have been threatened with weapons. An earlier (1992) study found that 8.4% of women had been threatened with weapons, and 6.9% had suffered armed violence.

The most recent study, by the Citizen Security Division of the Ministry of the Interior,[5] shows that during the second trimester of 2002, domestic violence was the fourth most frequently reported offence at national level, with a total of 32,515 reported cases. This represents a 12.3% increase over the figures for the same trimester last year.

Political and economic marginalisation of women

For Chilean social scientist Humberto Maturana, violence has its origins in the denial of the other person's truth in order to obtain obedience and subjection. A milieu of "conquerors" and "conquered," where some people or groups have the truth and others do not, promotes violence in relationships.

This process of annulling or destroying the adversary constitutes, in Maturana's opinion, the origin of violence. The imposition of "certainties" and disqualification of views that are different, often by force, has served as the basis for cultural, political, economic, and gender models in Chile.[6]

In Chile women did not obtain their right to vote, and thereby acquire citizen status, until 1947. As to participation in public office, women comprise only 11.5% and 5% of the total number of members elected to the House of Representatives and Senate, respectively. By the end of 1999, women barely amounted to 35% of the workforce, and as late as 2000 women were receiving an average income corresponding to 67.5% of the income of men.[7]

A cultural feature that has a direct effect on domestic violence is patriarchy. Men construct their identities around a model that gives them a mandate to provide, compete and win. Women, on the other hand, have been culturally assigned the role of being passive and obedient; this is seen as an extension of women's "natural" responsibilities within the domestic sphere, such as motherhood. These social stereotypes hinder women's holistic development and make them financially dependent on their spouses.

Violence begets violence

Discrimination and violence are also, in large measure, behaviours learned early in childhood. In homes where violent relationships prevail, both sons and daughters tend to reproduce this phenomenon in their own families and environment. According to a recent UNICEF study, one factor bearing on the abuse of children and in the reproduction of this behaviour in society is the existence of violence between parents.[8] For example, 70% of women who were physically abused said that these incidents took place in front of their children. Violence between parents inevitably creates harmful psychological effects in children.

Yet domestic violence and its profound discrimination and abuse are usually hidden – invisible in private life – and its victims muzzled.

Aída's story

I lost my mother when I was five. My father remarried, and soon after I began to be abused by my stepmother – both very much abused and marginalised. I had to get up around five or six o'clock in the morning to sweep the chicken coop, look after the garden, stoke the fire – we used coal for fire – put the kettle on to boil, do this, do that, a whole lot of things. I then knocked on her door to waken her, only to get a hard piece of bread to eat for breakfast. At the same time, this woman had a son my same age. She had a *trinche* (locked cupboard) in the house where she kept fresh milk, condensed milk, cheese, eggs...all for her son.

All of this I had to endure. I'm not making up a story from something I read from Cinderella. I had to run when I saw her coming, to place some cushions down where she was going to sit, had to really treat her like a queen. That's just the way things were.

My father used to tell this woman that as long as she left our eyes and mouths untouched, the rest didn't matter. So she would hit me, because I was the youngest and because I was always *súper pará* (quick to react and stand up for myself). Not only did my stepmother hit me, but my older brothers also had the authority to beat me. In fact, I have a very clear memory of my brother: once, he saw me talking with a boy on the street and he slapped me on the face, with his open hand, and left me there, bleeding. I've had to see it all and cry for everything in life. That's what makes one ready to face anything that could come along.

I used to shine this woman's shoes. One day, while I was shining her shoes she was berating me. I suddenly reacted and thought: what would she do if I threw the shoes at her? And I did it! She beat the *miechica* (pulp) out of me, but I felt liberated. I always remember feeling – even much later in life when my husband would beat me – that this wouldn't last for-

ever, that things would change.

Years later I came to Santiago when I was 14 years old. All my siblings were in this city as well as aunt of mine; she had seen how things were for me and sent for me as soon she could. While in Santiago, I met this 17-year-old guy. He would come up to me looking like a prince, well dressed, really '*encachaito*' (handsome). He chased me and chased me until he got what he wanted.

We met at a party, on 18 September.[9] There wasn't anyone who could get him off my back; he was like a disease. He would wait for me outside work; I couldn't get rid of him. We hadn't been courting for even a month when he raped me; it was like being assaulted. He had been telling me that nothing bad would ever happen to me. Almost immediately he changed and told me to have sexual intercourse, willingly or unwillingly, otherwise he would tear my clothes off. It was something tragic for me, at my age (15 years old).

Afterwards he said he had done it because he loved me – that if he hadn't done it like that, he never would have gotten me and that he needed to have a woman. But the fact that he had taken me by force left a mark on me forever. Because the only thing I could say after that was "yes, yes, yes." I felt terrible when he would say to me "don't worry, I'll talk with your brothers." He asked for my hand in marriage when he had already raped me.

Before we got married, that is during the time a couple wait for their wedding date to be set and all that, he had started to hit me. Any reason would do. Say, for example, that we were to meet at seven o'clock in the evening. If for one reason or another I didn't arrive at or before seven, he beat me. Or any other reason would do. If a fly buzzed around, he would hit me immediately. Afterwards he would act hurt to the core and would do things for me. I was so stupid that I believed it all and would even give him massages so he wouldn't leave me.

I then got married, already pregnant, and looked for a room to rent. I always led the way. That was the mistake I made. It's because I'm from the South. For me, it was my responsibility to find somewhere to live. I bought two cups, two plates, pans, and everything else two people need. He found that he could leave me with all the responsibilities. But to him, I was a *huasita* (derogatory term used for women) – that's how he always treated me, saying I was stupid and that this was why he had to go out.

Sometimes he would tell me we were going to go out somewhere, and since he never took me anywhere I would get all fixed up. Yet when I was ready he would pretend to be tired and lie down, or he would begin to make love to me and we would end up not going anywhere. I feel he did anything he wanted to with me. The beatings increased. I tried to leave him several times, but I always had to go back. The last time he split my lip and a tooth came loose. I was always covered with bruises. His mother would say to me, "When he hits you, it isn't because of what he's saying. He hits you because he's jealous." When I was menstruating, this man pretty much wanted to throw me out of the house, because he wouldn't accept the fact that he couldn't use me.

They beat you so much, so much, that they make you believe you are insignificant; you end up believing it.

Even so, in spite of all the bad things that were happening to me, I helped other people. I'd find children roaming the streets and I would give them food and take them to the shelters. I took a first aid course and would go to give people their shots at the top of the hill, and I wouldn't charge for it.

The priests would tell me I had a twofold look: that I looked with my soul and with my heart. At church I discovered who I was, what my life had been and what my initial relationship with my husband was. I discovered and understood I had been raped and that I had married my rapist. The man who hit me so much and looked for ways to punish me was

wrong, because he didn't have the right to do that. When I understood all this and began to grow, it was horrible because a war took place between us.

The church helped me to grow, to develop, but... with my job and the money I began to make, I was finally able to leave the man that beat me. One day he followed me and got into the same *micro* (bus) as I. When I saw him, I felt the same fear, the same panic as when he would hit me. It was unusual that I was alone, because my children are always protecting me. He sat down behind me and began to talk filth.

I was very scared, but I said to myself, "I promised myself I would turn him in, so I'm going to get off and do that as soon as we get to the street of the police station." The bus stopped and I got off, and he got off right behind me, whispering things in my ear. So I said to him, "Are you coming with me? I'm going to turn you in." After that came all the legal proceedings and now, well, I'm more at ease now.

My biggest supporters were my children. I have given them all the love I never received. The same is true with my grandchildren. I've given them everything I had kept inside. That is what gives me purpose in life. People listen to me and believe what I say and what I do, because every last thing is a testimony about life, about a life situation. For me, every process I have had to go through has been important, because I've tried to take advantage of it all for all those people that expect so much from us.

Progress towards change

It has been a long process in Chile and much remains to be done.

In the 1950s, the Government recognised women's issues as a public policy concern, and this led to assistance programs aimed at improving their living conditions and increasing child and family protection.

In the 1960s, policies aimed at women included the promotion of organisations that would open up spaces for women's participation in specific social issues; during the 1970s, state policies were channelled to women through these organisations. The active mobilisation of women's organisations and civil society has resulted in significant policy initiatives. In 1991 the National Service for Women (SERNAM), created by the Government to promote equal opportunities between men and women, and to guarantee the full exercise of the rights of women, was created. It has been a leading actor on the issue of intra-family violence, through various campaigns, programs and the creation of interdisciplinary networks at different political levels.

In a critical development in 1994, SERNAM enacted the *Law on Domestic Violence* (No. 19.325), which is discussed in more detail below. Subsequently, the *Plan for Equal Opportunities for Women* (1994–1999) was formulated. And in 1996, Chile signed the *Convention of Belem Do Pará* (Inter-American Convention on the Prevention, Punishment, and Eradication of Violence against Women) aimed at preventing and eradicating violence against women. These initiatives reflect the aspirations and struggle of diverse groups of women to ensure that women benefit from policymaking institutions and processes.

A law, but not enough

The 1994 *Law on Domestic Violence* (No. 19.325) is significant in that it:

- recognises the different types of physical, psychological, sexual and economic violence
- takes family violence out of the private sphere

and

- assigns it the category of an act punishable by law.

The latter point alone represents enormous progress: prior to the *Law on Domestic Violence* (LDV), the serious situation of abuse within the family was not considered a punishable offence.

Two other aspects of the LDV deserve highlighting. The first is the range of people to whom it applies:

any man, woman or child affected by domestic violence can file a complaint, and the law applies even if the person who committed the violence no longer lives with the family. The second is its measures towards protecting the physical or psychological integrity of the injured woman and her family as well as her livelihood and patrimony, and to facilitate due legal process to ensure a swift solution to the complaint.

Once the LDV was enacted, the number of complaints filed by women increased significantly. In 1994 there had only been 1,419 domestic violence complaints filed in Chile; in 1996 this figure jumped to 57,939.[10] This proved the expectations that existed regarding the possibility of finding swift and concrete solutions to situations of violence.

In spite of this progress, implementation of the LDV has revealed a number of limitations that need to be urgently corrected. For example, it privileges the married couple as a unit over the protection of the woman; this understanding exerts pressure for some type of reconciliation between the parties. To date, judges have rarely used the protective measures contemplated under the LDV. Also, a lack of adequate supervision makes it difficult to ensure compliance with preventive measures, such as prohibiting, restricting or limiting the presence of the offender in the home, or limiting or prohibiting the offender from appearing at the injured party's workplace.

The recent SERNAM study highlights that

- statistically, it takes an average of seven years for a woman to make her first official complaint – hence the importance of facilitating women's access to justice through networks of different institutions

and that

- although over 70% of the people who make use of juridical services are women, mostly because of violence in the family, only one out of four women suffering serious violence has asked for help from the courts.

Shortcomings in the LDV mean that those who inflict abuse may not necessarily be punished. Unfortunately, as the Citizen Security Division of the Ministry of the Interior report highlights, even when the number of reports increase, the number of arrests are still very few. This is partly due to the level of familiarity people have with this form of aggression.

It is also because, in most cases, the aggressor is the husband or the father. Abused women or their children make the complaint, but they do not complete the legal process because they fear the consequences. Economic dependence on the aggressor leads thousands of women to keep on accepting mistreatment. In most cases, a woman who is a victim of abuse does not want her spouse to be deprived of his freedom, so as to not to jeopardise their family income. In other cases, the injured party feels guilt for causing her own predicament, or decides to tolerate the abuse as a normal way of relating in the family.

Currently, some amendments to the LDV are being discussed in the Chamber of Deputies; these are aimed at providing greater protection for the integrity of victims and those who report the incidents. Among a number of proposed changes is the creation of Family Courts: the idea is that these more specialised courts will replace the juvenile courts that are currently used to handle such cases, and facilitate better access to the justice that is inherent in the Laws on Domestic Violence, Paternity and Food Alimony.

Dealing with the causes

The LDV has clearly drawn attention to the phenomenon of domestic violence, and helped raise awareness among broad segments of the population. This is a solid beginning. However, its measures essentially address the symptoms and not the cause of the problem.

The fact is that the structural conditions for social inequality persist, impairing fundamental rights and potentially generating violence. One of these is women's lack of access to education. In a study carried out by SERNAM, researchers verified that as their level of education increases, women are less likely to live in a violent relationship. The prevalence of physical and/or sexual violence is 40% among women with an incomplete basic or middle-level education,

whereas for those who have completed their high school education it is 29.1%, and for those who have completed university education, incidence of violence drops to 28.5%.[11]

Civil society initiatives

There remains a need to develop initiatives that focus on the preventive and educational spheres. Along these lines, in July 2001 SERNAM and over 70 other civil society organisations carried out a campaign to reduce violence within families, under the theme "*No dejes que la violencia golpee a tu pareja* (Don't let violence hit you as a couple)." The hope is that this is the beginning of a process of reflection that will advance to build a culture of peace in Chilean families and society, where every man and woman can enjoy the same rights and responsibilities.

With the participation of a range of civil society actors, SERNAM has led the formulation of a new *Plan of Equal Opportunities for Men and Women* for the 2000–2010 period.

Another recent SERNAM campaign is the Protect Network, which was initiated by President Lagos in recognition of the need for a stronger, more coordinated response from both private and public sectors to detect and prevent intra-family violence, child mistreatment and sexual abuse. The Protect Network's main objective is to encourage the active participation of civil society in preventing these problems. Various public services and representatives of social organisations, such as professional colleges, student federations, church groups, NGOs and religious communities, together make up this campaign.

The Church

Churches in Chile have been active in the struggle against domestic violence. During the military dictatorship period, the church opened avenues for the expression of people's concerns that were prohibited by the military regime. Many solidarity and personal growth initiatives appeared and were developed under the protection of the church. When democratic governance returned, these initiatives found ways to advance independent of the church, but churches remain active in trying to curb violence against women. The Roman Catholic Church, for example, deals with domestic abuse from both the individual spiritual side and by strengthening of the family through preventive approaches.

World Vision Chile

Although the issue is a complex one, World Vision believes that violent behaviour that threatens the basic rights of men, women and children, can be changed through mobilising and involving civil society. There is still much to be done to eliminate prejudices and help create relationships based upon respect within Chilean society, but the changes that have taken place to date allow for a more optimistic view. For example, thanks to the campaigns carried out by both the Government and NGOs, the incidence of serious physical violence against children was reduced by 26% between 1994 and 2000. And the introduction of the Law on Domestic Violence has placed this issue firmly on the agenda and helped raise the awareness of wide sectors of the population.

World Vision has actively participated in various campaigns led by SERNAM, most recently joining the Protect Network publicly in organising a walk for the rights of children. More than one thousand children from different World Vision Area Development Program projects participated in this walk. They were received at the Presidential Palace by the Minister for the Interior, Heraldo Muñoz; the Minister for the National Service for Women, Adriana Delpiano; and the Director of the National Service for Minors, Delia del Gatto.

Violence is not an isolated issue. Plans and programs require people learning to relate better with each other, meeting and accepting each other's differences, and working together in an organised way. For this reason, we believe the organisation of society plays a fundamental role in creating spaces of encounter, training and prevention for families, and actions for the protection of victims.

Various World Vision projects now include modules on domestic violence as part of their training programs. In addition, they encourage the active participation of other institutions in providing different workshops and conferences.

Another element that allows us to look more optimistically at the future is the series of programs that have as their objective the holistic development of the family – with the active participation of both parents and their children. The family is a strategic space where transforming models and new forms of relationships can be sustainably established. Within this space, World Vision Chile works on both promoting the rights of children and women, and on strengthening relationships between couples through retreats that allow sharing and reflection. These projects have yielded very good results, considerably improving relationships between many partners.

A more structural issue related to violence is that of poverty. Resentment, lack of opportunities, illiteracy and drugs are factors that help create conditions for violent relations. World Vision implements economic development plans and programs that aim at improving the quality of life of people, their families and the community as a whole. Within this approach, we seek to create more egalitarian relations within the family, since many cases of violence occur due to economic dependency, where the breadwinner holds the power. When both spouses earn money, the issue becomes less problematic.

Closing

Domestic violence in Chile is a critical issue that particularly affects women, but is causing concern in broad sectors of society. There are many cultural elements that reinforce the use of violence and that reproduce it as a way of resolving conflict.

The enactment of the *Law on Domestic Violence* is a useful first step. However, the situation in Chile continues to be critical. The actions promoted by the National Service for Women (SERNAM) have led the Government to consider the nexus of problems that affect women, among them violence, and include integrated solutions to these problems in national priorities.

In addition to the necessary protective measures and punishments contained in the *Law on Domestic Violence*, new formative actions are needed so that, one step at a time, there can be progress in building a culture of peace. Violence is a learned behaviour, to which children are socialised by the family. It is here where cultural patterns and forms of relating are learned that, although violent, are accepted as normal. It is common for adult perpetrators of violence to have been abused in their own childhoods. In order to effectively deal with violence within the family, a multi-disciplinary approach is needed that includes different actors and levels of action.

Violence in the family marks those who experience it: women, the main people affected, show low self-esteem, depression and isolation. Therefore not only legal assistance, but also psychological and social support are needed for the victims.

Perpetrators of domestic violence, on the other hand, have few resources at hand to help them overcome this problem. Plans and programs are needed that concentrate on the individual man, on his capacities and potential, and that help to rebuild dignity, promote reflection, bringing new knowledge and development tools, and strengthening values.

It has taken long periods of struggle and mobilisation to promote the elimination of, and to raise the awareness of society and its institutions regarding, violence within families. Our task in the future is not an easy one, but neither is it hopeless, as it might have seemed in the past. The community is now quite aware of the seriousness of the problem of violence within society. Programs, both by the Government as well as those by other NGOs, and that follow similar lines to those of World Vision Chile, have made a real difference to women and families suffering from this problem.

World Vision Chile has joined the efforts to build a culture in which peace and well-being become both the ends and the means of transforming relationships founded on violence and discrimination into more equitable ones based on mutual respect. We strongly believe that if we continue to follow the path we have taken, violence can be eradicated from the coming generations of Chileans.

References

[1] Ms. Moreno is a counsellor for the Fundación para la Superación de la Pobreza (Foundation to Overcome Poverty). In 1999, she was designated "Illustrious Daughter" by the Municipality of Renca. In March 2001, the Metropolitan Intendance honoured her, as part of the government events to celebrate International Women's Day, and she received an award from the First Lady, Luisa Durán, for her contributions as a People's Woman Leader.

[2] Centro de Análisis de Políticas Públicas (Public Policy Analysis Centre), *Detection and Analysis of the Prevalence of Domestic Violence, Metropolitan Region* (in Spanish), Universidad de Chile, Santiago, 2001. Most women who are physically or sexually violated are also victims of psychological abuse.

[3] Soledad Larraín, *Study on the Prevalence of Domestic Violence and Condition of Women in Chile* (in Spanish), 1992.

[4] Centro de Análisis de Políticas Públicas, *op. cit.*

[5] División de Seguridad Ciudadana del Ministerio del Interior de Chile, *Informe Semestral y Trimestral de estadísticas nacionales sobre denuncias y detenciones por delitos de mayor connotación social y violencia intrafamiliar*, Santiago, first quarter 2002, second quarter April–June 2002.

[6] Humberto Maturana, "La exigencia niega la legitimidad del otro," in *El sentido de lo humano*, Dolmen Ediciones, Santiago, 2000, p. 37.

[7] Ministerio de Planificación y Cooperación (Ministry of Planning and Cooperation), *Study on the Situation of Women in Chile*, Santiago, October 2001; and Women's National Service Database http://www.sernam.gov.cl/estadisticas/. Interestingly, the more education women have, the greater the discrepancy between the salaries of men and women. The Ministry study found that women with 0–3 years of schooling receive 18.6% less income than men with the same level of education, whereas women who completed 13 or more years of education received only 51.5% of the salary of men with comparable schooling.

[8] UNICEF, *Comparative Study on Child Abuse, 1994 and 2000.*

[9] Chilean Independence Day

[10] Domestic Violence Complaints Office of the Santiago Court of Appeals, *Annual Figures on Domestic Violence in Chile* (in Spanish), http://www.fundaciónpobreza.cl/violencia/antecedentes generales/

[11] Centro de Análisis de Políticas Públicas, *op. cit.*

The links between HIV/AIDS and violence: Towards a dialogue with men

Sekai Nzenza Shand

Introduction

World Vision HIV and AIDS campaigns have encouraged prevention methods, such as "A, B and small c" (Abstinence outside of marriage, Being faithful within marriage, and condom use for people who cannot or will not practice self-discipline). Somehow forgotten is that traditional rural women have little power to implement ABc or other programs designed to curb HIV/AIDS.

Regardless of race, economic, political or social status, all women are at risk of experiencing sexual violence. Sexual violence refers to the sexual imposition of unwanted force through threats or physical coercion. This form of abuse against women is not only both a psychological and physical aberration, but also a shocking violation of women's basic rights.

In the past, HIV/AIDS and sexual violence were researched separately from various perspectives. Research on the relationship between violence and HIV infection is still scarce. But incidences of rape and sexual coercion show that violence against women does have links to HIV/AIDS. As the prevalence of HIV infection among women escalates, sexual violence should be treated with even more serious concern. It is abuse that has adverse consequences for a woman's sexual and reproductive health and the well-being of her children. NGOs (non-governmental organisations), community organisations and policy-makers should recognise that violence against women has serious negative impacts on development.

As HIV/AIDS continues to spread throughout Southern Africa, the need to protect women and to encourage men to change their sexual behaviours is a matter of urgency. In South Africa, for example, sexual violence is increasingly responsible for HIV infections. A growing number of women are being sexually exploited and murdered. Women who are subject to sexual violence live with the fear, or the reality, of having contracted HIV.

The major objective of this paper is to explore the disempowerment of women and their vulnerability to violence and to HIV transmission. In particular, it is highlighted that:

- Power structures, gender inequalities and traditional views of sexuality are an impediment to halting HIV transmission rates. Other factors exacerbating the situation include poverty; urban migration (severe economic hardships fuelled by the disparity between the city and countryside create an environment enabling the virus to spread); and violence against women.
- Some NGO messages about preventive methods have been misplaced, irrelevant or inapplicable to the cultural contexts of women and men in rural areas of Africa. Interventions were based on the assumption that, given informed choice, African women can control when, how and with whom they engage in sex. For example, the promotion of condoms alone in rural areas has not been effective in halting the epidemic. Although in some places condoms may be accessed cheaply at local shops and health centres, there remain social, economic and cultural barriers prohibiting women from using condoms. World Vision and other NGOs now recognise HIV/AIDS as a disease of inequality and marginalisation. In Southern Africa, we seek to promote gender equality in programs and to provide access to education and resources.
- By excluding men from interventions, HIV/AIDS programs have inadvertently failed to prevent men from inflicting violence on women.

- Finally, recommendations are presented for WorldVision and other NGOs and practitioners working in HIV/AIDS prevention, care, treatment and advocacy.

Mai Esther's story

For over 20 years, my extended family had gathered to celebrate Christmas. Each year, we noticed that another family member was missing. So far, those missing and buried were relatively young.

Two years ago, my sister Constance was buried. She was 48 and a mother of two teenage girls. Last Christmas, my sister-in-law Esther was missing. We thanked God that she was not dead – she was nursing her 62-year-old mother. The family still gathered, as they have always done. Esther's mother was too old to die from AIDS, my mother told her friends. After all, my aunt was a public health specialist working in prisons. At her age, she would have known about AIDS and she could not have died from the disease.

We missed Esther and we prayed for her mother. I remembered seeing Esther's mother at the village church last Christmas holidays. Mai Esther (Esther's mother) was the leader of the women's group. I recall her singing beautifully, in her Anglican Mothers' white blouse, black skirt and blue coloured headdress. She prayed that God would spare the lives of our young from the deadly AIDS virus.

This year, on the third of January, Mai Esther's uniform was decked neatly on her coffin. The women from the Anglican Mothers group gathered in the working-class suburb of Chitungwiza, Harare. All night they sang around her coffin. At four in the morning, I offered Esther a cup of tea and we took a break away from the mourners. We sat in the lounge room. On the mantelpiece was a photo of Esther's parents, both of them smiling. The father, Jonasi, was wearing a nice suit and tie. Esther recalled how she had nursed her father until he died three years before. "After this funeral, I shall cut my father's face from the photo," said Esther. I asked why. "Because, if it was not for him, my mother would be alive. I must avenge the violence done to my mother. She was too old to die from AIDS," Esther cried.

Esther was angry and so was I. Mai Esther was a good rural woman, a respected grandmother, leader of her church, counsellor and caregiver of the sick. She was looking after five children orphaned as a result of HIV/AIDS. She was also a good farmer, a gifted singer and dancer deeply rooted in the cultural traditions of her Shona culture. She respected her husband and did not question his faithfulness when he came home three times a year. Husbands leave home to work in the city; wives stay at home, care for children and work in the fields. This was the practice and still is. Sometimes it was natural that a man took a mistress in the city. If the relationship produced children, the young mistress became a wife and settled in the village, next door to the senior wife. At first there are tensions and jealousy. But gradually the two women accept each other and stay home to care for their children in the absence of the father. This is considered normal. When the husband returns home and demands sex from his wives, they must submit. It's considered to be his right: after all, he paid the bride price for them. He can physically assault them if they do not grant him his rights. Shona society has done this for generations. The village people will tell you that this cannot be changed overnight. Even HIV/AIDS cannot quickly change behaviour.

We buried Mai Esther back home in the village. She had a good funeral. This coming Christmas, we pray that no more among us will be missing. Meanwhile, young girls in the village pray that eligible men from the city do not bring home the virus. Yet we now know that they will bring it. Our anger will continue to rise, as we bury yet another family member. We are angry with Jonasi and with all men like him. For some time now, we have blamed them for their power over women and the infliction of physical and emo-

tional violence on women.

The following day I set off to do some research on women, HIV and violence, already predisposed to the notion that African men recklessly and knowingly inflict women with violence and are largely responsible for the high HIV infection rate in women. Mai Esther's story and those of others confirmed my theory.

After two weeks of interviewing rural women and commercial sex workers, I was struck by the lack of male voices in my study. I went back to Esther's family. I wanted to know whether Jonasi had any regrets about his treatment of women before he died.

Traditional poverty and power: a web of vulnerability

Vulnerability of girls

In the past, young girls in Zimbabwe, Malawi and Mozambique received sex education from senior aunts and other elderly women. Even where sex education is taught in schools, girls do not have access to information on the mechanics of HIV or STD (sexually transmitted disease) transmission and prevention because elders do not understand the disease. In any case, most rural girls leave school before they fully gain an understanding of reproductive health. Without education or skills, girls become more economically dependent on men. Young women who marry wealthy older men ("sugar daddies") have less power – often becoming second wives – and are more vulnerable to violent abuse if they "disobey." Some end up as commercial sex workers in the event of a marriage break-up.

In romantic relationships generally, girls are sometimes coerced into sex to "prove" that they love the man. Men have more sexual freedom than women. Unfaithfulness is regarded as "normal" in men but is seen as unacceptable in women. In the Tete province of Mozambique, for example, women are expected to preserve their virginity until marriage while young men are encouraged to gain sexual experience through experimentation. Young men compete to have sex with as many virgins as they can seduce. The masculine identity of men who fail to meet the required number of virgins is usually questioned. As a result, in order to prove their masculinity, young men go to the extent of raping young women.

Petrosi

During a recent visit to South Africa, I asked my taxi driver, Petrosi, to tell me about the increasing stories of men who rape women in Johannesburg. First, he laughed, then said:

"I am a Zulu man, a warrior. I do not rape women. Why should I? Men with little power do that. I have plenty of power so I do not rape. I only beat my wife and my girlfriend when they disobey. Men who rape are cowards and there are many of us around. It's the young people who are doing it when the women refuse to obey… I am a good man. I pay rent, feed the children, so women must obey me because I am the man."

His girlfriend or second wife, Jane, sat next to him and smiled, shaking her head.[1]

While traditionalists like Petrosi believe they have the right to punish "disobedient" women, other men simply seek women out for the purposes of rape. In post-apartheid South Africa, a woman is raped every minute. [2] Johannesburg has been called the "rape capital" of the world. The high incidence of rape of young girls is attributed to the myth that a man who is HIV-positive will be cured if he has sex with a virgin. Yet the South African Government will not sanction provision of anti-AIDS drugs to these women, girls and children.[3]

In urban Zimbabwe today, sexual abuse of girls is increasing and is one of the most violent forms of child exploitation. As in rural Mozambique, there is a double standard: the same girls are expected to be virgins at marriage; a man can beat his new bride

if he discovers that she is not a virgin. Village girls are expected to be subservient and ignorant about sex, as they wait for the right man.

Clearly, HIV prevention and education should target both young men and women.

Traditional attitudes and practices

In many cultures, there are restrictions based on age or gender regarding access to information about sexuality. For example, in traditional Shona society, only uncles or grandparents can discuss sex with male adolescents; similarly, it is the role of the aunt to instruct the young niece about sexual conduct. Virginity was regarded as a personal and community virtue. Although sexually transmitted diseases existed, communities had traditional methods to cure them.

Teachers in schools and other institutions working with adolescents are concerned about providing sex education for fear of breaking down the cultural norms and therefore "encouraging" the young to engage in premarital sex. HIV/AIDS has presented communities with new challenges.

The risk of HIV infection also increases as a result of female genital mutilation, and traditional sex practices such as "dry" sex,[4] which results in tearing and bleeding during intercourse. Forms of rape also multiply the risk of HIV infection.

Other traditional practices are also causing an increasing risk of HIV infection. For example, in the event of a man dying from AIDS, his surviving brother can inherit his young wife. Similarly, an unmarried sister or niece can inherit her late sister's husband to enable her to care for the children. Refusal to comply with the practice can result in the woman being ostracised or physically abused.

Quite often, women do not know that they have sexually transmitted diseases because symptoms are hard to detect until the condition becomes more serious. Furthermore, interviews with women at two health centres in Zimbabwe show that women give priority to all other responsibilities and pay less attention to their own health.

In other parts of Southern Africa, traditional practices such as female genital mutilation (though not as widespread) and beauty tattooing when performed in non-sterile conditions can lead to HIV infection.

Rural poverty, economic dislocation

Migration to cities disrupts traditional rural families by separating men from their wives. This dislocation increases the risk of disease, as urban male migrants find new sex partners during long periods away from home. Similarly, truck drivers are vulnerable to contracting and spreading HIV due to the nature of their work.

Power to negotiate

Men have power and control over women. Traditional attitudes defining men's dominant roles in society place women in vulnerable positions.

Even women who have knowledge and awareness of HIV/AIDS, quite often do not succeed in negotiating condom use. For many women, asking men to use condoms is difficult because condoms are often associated with promiscuity, unfaithfulness and immoral behaviour. In fact, asking a man to use a condom often leads to adverse and violent reactions. Suggesting condom use in an existing relationship is almost impossible, because it raises issues of infidelity from both parties. Clearly, most women cannot initiate condom use for fear of risking violent indignation and abuse.

Even a woman like Mai Esther, with grown-up children and authority as a community leader who considered herself to be a moral Christian woman, could not have stopped her husband from sleeping with her even if she suspected that he might have HIV. Indeed, refusing him sex or asking him to use condoms might have suggested that she had engaged in extramarital sexual activity in his absence. One day, Mai Esther did have the courage to ask him to use a condom during one of his visits. He reacted with anger and beat her, before abandoning her in favour of the second wife. Because people with the virus appear healthy for some years, Jonasi did not know that he was infected. Without access to testing, most men do not know that they are infected – and that they need to protect their wives from it.

Male resistance to condom use and women's inabil-

ity to negotiate safer sex places women (as well as men) at greater risk of HIV infection.

Why do men inflict violence on women?

There are a wide range of factors contributing to male violence. Some common reasons include:

- history of abuse in one's own background as a child
- witnessed abuse of a family member
- knowledge and anger about one's HIV status
- use of drugs or alcohol
- fear or insecurity of losing one's masculine identity

Why are women silent?

The same fear of violence that prevents women from asking men to use condoms also limits their capacity to seek HIV/AIDS counselling and testing. In this regard, health professionals should consider the implications of encouraging women to reveal HIV infection to their partners. Disclosing one's HIV status can lead to accusations of unfaithfulness leading to domestic violence. Without adequate counselling and follow-up, victims of violence live in fear and have difficulty adhering to HIV treatment and procedures.

Similarly, pregnant women who test positive to HIV fear ostracism and domestic violence if they reveal their status. Since breast-feeding is regarded as the norm by most African societies, stigmatisation and abuse affect HIV-infected women who have been advised to feed their babies infant formula, if possible, to avoid mother-to-child transmission. In truth, infant formula is not an option for most African women due to unsafe water, unavailability of infant formula or poverty. Under these conditions WorldVision and the World Health Organisation (WHO) advise women to breast feed, knowing that there is a possibility that some children will become infected with HIV.[5]

The dilemma of informed choice

A common Western assumption is that women can assume responsibility for the prevention of HIV and violence once they know what the choices are. Informed choice is indeed a possibility in societies such as Australia or Western Europe where women have resources and know their rights. Many educational resources published in women's magazines talk about the right of women to make an informed choice, whether this is about breastfeeding, treatment, surgery or contraceptives. But most rural African women cannot control how and when they can engage in sexual activity. Their vulnerability to HIV infection increases as a result of their lack of educational opportunities, economic dependence on men, poverty, sexual exploitation, violence and rape.

Constance

Constance sat on the veranda of a dusty shop at Domboshava, 50 kilometres northeast of Harare, the capital of Zimbabwe. Her face was swollen and there were dry cracks of blood on her nose. Local market women sat around her. She talked freely and openly about how she was assaulted by a soldier the previous night.

"I refused to have sex without a condom and he hit me. First, he used fists, and then he hit me on the head with the barrel of his gun," she said. The women shook their heads and said that Constance should have known better than taking on a soldier as a customer for the night. "But the soldiers from the DRC (Democratic Republic of Congo) have money. They normally pay on the spot," said Constance. "I need to feed my two children back in the village."

For the rest of the evening, I sat with the market women and commercial sex workers (CSWs) at Domboshava. CSWs aged 19 to 45 told varied stories of violence and abuse they experienced during the course of their work.

Most women do not freely choose to be commercial sex workers. Some are forced into prostitution. For others at Domboshava Growth Point, it is a choice they make to survive and save their children from starvation.

But such choices are risky, as demonstrated by the violence women like Constance experience. The women's ability to exercise choice is limited.

In rural areas, social norms limit access to information about sexual matters. Most village women accept the high-risk sexual behaviour of husbands and are exposed to infection. Mai Esther epitomises the role of most rural women – powerless when faced with male demands. When her husband became violent, she "accepted" this norm. Jonasi ignored a crucial responsibility to change his behaviour. But how much knowledge of HIV/AIDS did he have?

Exclusion of men from mainstream programming

In rural Zimbabwe, as noted above, young men are expected to be promiscuous before marriage. Among young male adults who are sexually active, sex is usually unplanned and occurs frequently. School leavers engage in sex more as a pastime out of boredom, putting themselves at greater risk of contracting STDs including HIV/AIDS. Generally, by the time young men get married, they have engaged in sexual intercourse with at least ten girls.[6]

Yet, due to their limited knowledge of these diseases, most young men engaging in sexual intercourse are unaware of the consequences of their actions to their partners and to themselves. Furthermore, many young men are unlikely to visit a health centre seeking preventive material as they find the experience embarrassing. Only recently have health centres in Zambia and Zimbabwe reserved spaces where youth can discuss sexual matters and ask for condoms in private.

In rural-based societies these young men, like their fathers, control the structures of power over women, which means they have an important role to play in bringing about behaviour change. This gives men the opportunity to understand that their change in attitudes and behaviour can bring positive results, and influence the way HIV is spread.

What strategies have World Vision and other NGOs used to address men?

Women and development: historical background

> Gender inequality is a fundamental driving force of the AIDS epidemic and therefore must be addressed centrally in responding to the epidemic.[7]

It is a truism to say that during the 1980s, NGOs and governments underestimated the potential magnitude of HIV/AIDS in Africa. Experts believed that the heterosexual aspect of the pandemic would be halted if high-risk "transmitters" – such as commercial sex workers, truck drivers and single people likely to engage in sex with multiple partners – were comprehensively targeted. Condom use was encouraged but not emphasised.[8] As an example, World Vision's successful Uzumba, Maramba and Pfungwe integrated health, agriculture and child survival project (known as UMPHWA) in Zimbabwe hardly focused on HIV/AIDS. Women visiting the health centre for family planning purposes received some education on HIV/AIDS. But at the time, rural women were not considered at risk. It took us a decade to see the devastating effects of the disease in rural areas.

Generally, men were excluded from mainstream HIV programming. Reasons included assumptions that women were the most vulnerable to HIV because their power was much less than men's; in addition, women were reluctant to discuss sexual issues in the presence of men. World Vision worked with women in development for a number of years. In fact, World Vision and other NGOs have few development projects in Africa that focus on men.[9]

Yet by paying less attention to men, NGOs have inadvertently allowed violence against women to continue unchallenged. In the Inkoaranga project in Tanzania, as an example, World Vision focused on female sex workers and did not pay enough attention to their male clients. At Domboshava Growth Point in Zimbabwe, local health workers provide education and counselling to women seeking condoms or treatment for STDs. A survey of men seeking treatment at the health centre found that men believed women were responsible for illnesses to men. On

discovering that he was HIV-positive, one young man went back to the bar and severely assaulted a young woman he had never met before. "It's women like you who spread the virus," he said.

In Southern Africa, men are at the epicentre of the epidemic. Petrosi is too busy running a private taxi business to have direct access to HIV educational resources. Furthermore, his aggressive sense of manhood may deter him from seeking information. Stories such as those of Petrosi and Jonasi could easily create images of a stereotypical African male – selfish, controlling, inconsiderate, dominant and with violent and rapist tendencies. The sad result is that women bear the afflictions caused by men's actions. By the time a woman gets married, she is most likely already infected with HIV. Because a person can carry the virus and stay healthy for years, women usually discover their HIV status when they are pregnant or become ill after birth. Being ill and caring for an infected child places an enormous burden on women.

Interventions cannot be effective without men's involvement. In Zimbabwe, as we have seen, men have the power to make decisions to have sex with or without a condom; women know what is needed to protect themselves, but without the cooperation of men, they cannot succeed. Men will force their partners to submit.

NGO programs should not wait until it is too late to educate men and change their behaviours. It is important to include men in needs assessment interventions to understand their beliefs, views, perceptions and sexual practices.

Jonasi

When I inquired about Jonasi's character with the people closest to him during his illness, I was given an image of a most loving father and husband. His two wives and daughter had nursed him until he died in their arms at home. Jonasi spoke about his beliefs and sexual practices on his deathbed. "If I knew about this disease, I would not have engaged in sex outside my marriage," Jonasi had told his family.

He did not regret beating his wives: he was only doing what is expected of a male breadwinner in traditional Shona society. He did, however, apologise for inflicting violence in the form of a deadly disease on his two wives. Perhaps Jonasi was able to articulate his feelings because he was vulnerable and powerless.

It is clear that preventive education campaigns and policy makers did not reach Jonasi. They failed to provide Jonasi with the education and awareness he needed to protect his health and that of his family: he needed to know that he was engaging in risk taking behaviour by having multiple partners. Does he deserve our anger or our sympathy?

Ending violence toward women: strategic approaches

Recommendations

Programs seeking to end violence against women require a strategic and well-coordinated framework that includes many sectors of society at community, national and regional levels. They need to:

- train staff in development projects to focus on empowering women, and to recognise that violence is an unacceptable form of human rights violation
- in integrated health programs, view sexual violence as a major health problem
- at the program design stage, conduct gender-specific surveys to assess the level of violent abuse and build in structures to address it
- in communities that practise *lobola* or "bride price," teach men to understand that payment of this does not mean that a man "owns" the woman as his property; such a concept undermines the ability of a woman to leave a violent and abusive relationship
- focus advocacy initiatives on empowering women and girls, counselling and meeting the

needs of victims, liasing with government and other local institutions

- include youth and peer educators in HIV/AIDS programs
- seek to involve men and engage them in discussions to change community beliefs and attitudes about women and about how HIV/AIDS is spread; women cannot change sexual behaviour without the cooperation of men (see following section)
- improve girl children's access to formal schooling
- develop programs to teach girls about sexuality, AIDS, STDs and pregnancy; empower them with skills to refuse unwanted sex
- ensure that in development programs women have access to adequate health care and HIV/STD prevention services, while expanding voluntary HIV testing and counselling services
- provide women-friendly services; increase the availability of condoms in places where women are assured of confidentiality
- encourage more research into ways in which women can be empowered to put prevention into their own hands: for example, promote the use of the female condom and microbicides in order to prevent infection by HIV as well as other STDs
- support local women's groups and community organisations to create a dialogue with traditional leaders on issues of violence and HIV
- encourage education for boys and men that teaches them to respect girls and women; this way they can adopt responsible behaviours towards protecting themselves and their partners from HIV (see following section)

and

- promote and strengthen training opportunities for women through the provision of micro-credit and agricultural interventions; review lessons learned from successful projects and build upon existing structures.

Towards a dialogue with men

To date, World Vision's HIV/AIDS projects in Southern Africa aim to reduce levels of HIV-related risk behaviour through community-based education and awareness programs.

While women-only programs are important, excluding men can only continue to make women more vulnerable to HIV infection. Dissemination of family planning methods to men has largely been successful in Southern Africa: men were willing to listen to their wives and to health practitioners about having fewer children. Similar methods of educating men can bring about other behaviour changes. Currently, men have limited knowledge of the HIV virus; they do not necessarily approve of condoms particularly when they want to have children.

Educational interventions should begin by seeking men's willingness to engage in dialogue, then to approve and practice behaviour changes. Conversations with men suggest that many men have already gone through the stages of knowledge and approval and are now ready to adopt healthier sexual practices.[10]

In any given culture, masculine identity is constructed in diverse ways. Among the Masai, for example, a man could once prove his manhood by killing a lion. But with the scarcity of lions, Masai men seek other ways of defining masculinity. The fact that masculinities are subject to change over time indicates that, through advocacy, we can develop alternative versions of masculine identity that are conducive to preventing the spread of HIV infection.

This is an arena where the church can be effective. An increasing part of HIV prevention programs among youth is an emphasis on sexual abstinence before marriage. For example, in a recent trip to Zambia, I was amazed to see teens of both sexes openly speaking about abstinence. These youth were also sharing HIV education and awareness information with their non-Christian peers. Similar youth-led activities are widespread among congregations in Uganda. In South Africa, many churches are campaigning for abstinence before, and faithfulness within, marriage.

Inequality between men and women facilitates the transmission of HIV; therefore, a commitment to greater social and gender equality is a starting point in seeking to address the health of both women and men. At the same time, properly formulated strategies to include men's participation can help slow the spread of HIV/AIDS and other sexually transmitted diseases. Men who are aware of their responsibilities can also help prevent violence against women. NGOs should now build in new approaches to include men's participation in the design and implementation of AIDS prevention services.

Strategies to include men's participation

To reduce HIV transmission rates, prevention programs should seek better ways to dialogue with men in order to engage men to take responsibility for themselves and their partners. Education and communication at the grassroots are key to getting the message across to men. In developing strategic ways to give men important information on HIV and AIDS, programs might:

- develop messages in the mass media to specifically target men through radio, television and newspapers, and through video and pamphlets
- encourage use of celebrities and prominent people to speak out on issues surrounding HIV/AIDS, violence and discrimination
- target places where men gather and bring information to them; this could mean entering places such as bars, football matches and churches
- initiate a campaign based on audience analysis; research and monitor responses; and evaluate results
- promote the involvement of men in HIV prevention efforts
- increase resources and strengthen existing efforts
- review existing gender-focused programs and interventions and seek to include men in them

  (It is important, however, to assess whether the promotion of men's participation will disempower women; this is a legitimate risk, because men are already occupying positions of power and giving them attention could jeopardise women's access to knowledge and resources.)

and/or

- review current programs of prevention, health promotion and development and increase gender sensitivity and awareness

It is clear that, at a broader level, similar principles could be applied to NGO programs seeking to fight poverty, for example:

- include men in micro-enterprise projects

and

- encourage and promote men's role as farmers alongside women

Recommendations for advocacy: key principles

The President of World Vision International, Dean Hirsch, in his recognition and promotion of International Women's Day on 8 March 2002, announced:

> "World Vision is in a unique position to raise awareness of women's issues, advance gender equity, and create opportunities for dialogue and action. Our ministry seeks to follow Jesus Christ in his identification with the poor, the powerless, the afflicted, the oppressed, and the marginalised. God bestows equal dignity on all people, regardless of sex, age or condition."

- All women have the right to live in freedom without suffering from violence and abuse.
- Men, boys and the whole community have the responsibility to combat violence against women.
- Both men and women should have access to information and resources to allow the practice of responsible behaviour.
- While acknowledging and respecting social and

cultural diversity, there should be a universal approach to condemn sexual violence and to provide survivors with appropriate counselling and care.

Advocacy and programming

Clearly, while operational NGOs primarily focus on individual behaviour change, civil society institutions should also scale up policies and actions in order to reduce the spread of the epidemic. Recommendations for World Vision and other NGOs' advocacy and programming include:

- in partnership with World Vision's Gender Network, develop a World Vision Partnership-wide policy on HIV and sexual violence.
- through World Vision's Hope Initiative, advocate to promote an environment conducive to social change through the development of new partnership policies to combat HIV infection and violence against women (This can only be enhanced by scaling up HIV/AIDS advocacy and programming.)
- in collaboration with World Vision's Hope initiative,[11] develop systems and policies to support people experiencing sexual violence; encourage HIV testing and counselling for women, and safeguard confidentiality
- through community advocacy, develop resource materials/pamphlets for survivors of sexual violence and those at risk; resources should include information on the connections between HIV and sexual violence, the risks, HIV testing, and counselling procedures
- within HIV/AIDS programs, develop initiatives related to combating sexual violence; promote sharing of ideas through training of trainers, peer-support and focus groups, educational resource materials, seminars, forums and workshops
- through community development, include participation of traditional leaders, local government representatives, women's groups, churches, health workers, teachers and police services; liaise with other local groups and NGOs to initiate training programs related to HIV and sexual violence
- call for more research and systematic approaches to the integration of men
- include in program design efforts to counter discrimination and stigma associated with HIV/AIDS

and

- scale up efforts to challenge dominant and oppressive current norms responsible for violence against women and for causing an increase in the AIDS epidemic.

Closing

Today, the challenge is to develop strategies to involve men and increase their participation in ending violence against women. Clearly, women cannot change traditional attitudes without the support of men. While listening and responding to women's concerns, World Vision should design programmes with a specific intent to create opportunities for men to speak about their concerns. It is important that we seek to promote dialogue between men and women. In rural Southern Africa, encouraging men's participation has the potential to help communities understand the negative impact of violence and help them bring about behaviour change. Through direct interaction and participation, men can learn to acknowledge that violence and high-risk behaviours not only hurt women, they also negatively affect the fabric of society and undermine development.

Acknowledgement

I wish to thank staff and HIV/AIDS coordinators in World Vision Zimbabwe, Mozambique and South Africa for their support during the research for this paper. I also want to thank The Musasa Project, a women's refuge centre in Harare for access to their research and files. Above all, I want to acknowledge the openness of the women and men who were willing to share their personal stories, hoping that through dialogue, we can begin to address our problems without guilt or blame. There is hope in working together.

References

[1] Interview with Petrosi and Jane, Tembisa, South Africa, 17 January 2002.

[2] For a fuller account of men's role in increasing the spread of HIV/AIDS, see *South African Soccer*, December 2001/January 2002, Vol. 2, No. 6, pp. 72–74.

[3] A recent court order requires the government to provide nevirapine to reduce mother-to-child HIV infection.

[4] Avoidance of any lubricants, including the removal of vaginal secretions. Further background information including reasons for the practice can be found at: http://www.rho.org/html/hthps-b-02.html#drysex

[5] About 30–33% of HIV-infected women pass the disease to their children: roughly 60% of the time during pregnancy and birth and 40% through breast feeding. Concerning World Vision communities, Dr. Hector Jalipa relates that "If we take babies off breast milk and bottle-feed them, the rate of deaths would be around 60 per cent." Reported in Nigel Marsh, *Though HIV may be in Mothers' Milk, World Vision Africa Affirms the Breast*, Internal World Vision International communications document, November 1998.

[6] Interviews with ten men between the ages of 20 and 25 at Domboshava Growth Point, Zimbabwe, 2002.

[7] Peter Piot, Executive Director of the Joint United Nations Programme on HIV/AIDS (UNAIDS), http://www.unaids.org/index.html, 5 June 2000.

[8] Sekai Nzenza Shand, *Nkoaranga HIV/AIDS Review* (World Vision Australia in partnership with World Vision Tanzania), September 1995; and Tamara Kwarteng & Tim O'Shaughnessy, *Arumeru HIV/AIDS Prevention Project* (World Vision Australia), 1999, an evaluation report which has some excellent recommendations.

[9] An overview of HIV/AIDS prevention projects in East and Southern Africa show a strong focus on women. The truck drivers' project is, however, a good example of targeting men.

[10] Meetings with the male congregation at Jeche Primary School, Zimbabwe, 2002. Similarly, men in a Rwandan project at Gikongoro were very open to dialogue, September 2000.

[11] The Hope Initiative is a major World Vision programme with objectives of HIV/AIDS prevention, care for people affected by AIDS (such as people living with AIDS, their family members, and AIDS orphans), and advocacy for HIV/AIDS programming.

Commercial sexual exploitation of children: How extra-territorial legislation can help

Sara L. Austin

Introduction

Millions of boys and girls are trapped in sexual servitude, victims of what is rapidly becoming the most profitable criminal activity after drug trafficking. Whether this happens in their own homes and communities, or whether they are trafficked within their own country or across international borders, these children experience multiple forms of exploitation at the hands of those who seek to abuse them for sexual purposes. They experience physical, emotional, and psychological trauma, become vulnerable to contracting sexually transmitted diseases including HIV/AIDS, and are economically exploited. "It is painful to contemplate that, unlike illegal drugs, women and children are often sold again and again. Their abuse and pain are multiplied as the transactions increase." [1]

One key component to action against commercial sexual exploitation is legislative reform to criminalise these activities, to make it possible to prosecute offenders no matter where they commit such offences or where they currently reside. While legal action is only one means among many of addressing the problem, it is critical in helping create an international social and political climate where the commercial sexual exploitation of children will no longer be tolerated, and where there is no impunity for offenders. When implemented within the context of a comprehensive, multi-dimensional strategy to promote human rights, the enactment and enforcement of national and extra-territorial legislation against commercial sexual exploitation can be enormously effective in ensuring children's protection.

The intent of this paper is to draw greater attention to the actions taken by select countries to target commercial sexual exploitation of children through legislative reform. These countries have taken legal action against their own nationals who have committed sex offences abroad. Five countries in the developed world that have enacted extra-territorial legislation to halt the sexual exploitation of children[2] are highlighted.

The complex nature of gender-based violence, which certainly affects and exacerbates the commercial sexual exploitation of children, is briefly examined. This paper also highlights more broadly the need to protect children from all forms of sexual exploitation, as this in turn has a protective influence throughout their full life cycle in reducing their vulnerability to forms of commercial sexual exploitation.

Section 1 of this paper outlines both the scope and the nature of the problem, then examines the international social and legal context, and concludes with a detailed discussion of the need for strategic legal response to the commercial sexual exploitation of children. Section 2 provides case studies on five countries whose nationals commit sexual offences against children while abroad, outlining each nation's approaches to domestic and extra-territorial legislation, and highlighting strengths and weaknesses of their legal systems for addressing this problem as well as their success in implementation. A comparative analysis of those five countries follows. Section 3 provides conclusions and recommendations.

Section 1: Scope and nature of the problem

Determining the scope of commercial sexual exploitation of children has proven to be fraught with difficulty, in that the very nature of the crime typically keeps it hidden. Whether trapped in back rooms of brothels or massage parlours, hotel rooms or back alleys, these children remain invisible to the public. Those who control these children can thus continue to exploit them with reckless abandon.

Methods for estimating the number of children

trapped in the commercial sex industry, whether at the local, national, regional or global level, have varied greatly. Facts and figures are at best "approximate and anecdotal, calculated on the basis of the horror of field workers who have seen far too many children trapped in prostitution or suffering the consequences, and on the partial surveys and studies – all using different methodologies, sample bases and extrapolation formulae – that together show without a doubt that there are more than a million children caught in commercial sex, though (there is) little hope of ever knowing exactly how many."[3]

One of the most horrific implications of the absence of empirical data is that it has allowed governments to deny that this phenomenon exists within their boundaries,[4] thus compounding the obstacles to addressing the issue. The need for accurate and reliable data that is disaggregated by age and sex is absolutely critical in order to design strategic programmes and policies to eliminate commercial sexual exploitation of children.

In addition to the hidden nature of the problem, another complexity in measuring the scope of commercial sexual exploitation of children remains the myriad definitions of "child" and "commercial sexual exploitation". This paper uses internationally agreed-upon definitions: the term "child" (or children) refers to any person below the age of 18,[5] and the term "commercial sexual exploitation" refers to child prostitution, child pornography and trafficking of children for sexual purposes.[6]

International social context

Gender-based violence

The commercial sexual exploitation of children must be understood within an international social context that still tolerates and perpetuates gender-based violence. "Gender-based violence" is generally understood to be:

> ...an umbrella term for any harm that is perpetrated on a person against her/his will, and that has a negative impact on the physical and/or psychological health, development, and identity of the person. The violence is the result of gendered power relationships, determined by the social roles ascribed to males and females, almost always and across all cultures disparately impacting women and children. Violence may be physical, sexual, psychological, economic, or socio-cultural.[7]

A motivation and desire for power and domination is often at the root of gender-based violence,[8] so any efforts taken to combat the exploitation of children for sexual purposes must have at the very core of its strategy a plan to address the imbalance of power between men and women, and between adults and children. As such, strategies to address gender-based violence must seek to transform structures and systems that have typically disempowered women and children. Moreover, law enforcement bodies must be adequately equipped to deal with the gender dynamics of the commercial sexual exploitation of children, and the disproportionately high number of girls affected and male perpetrators.[9]

The *Declaration against Violence against Women*, adopted by the United Nations General Assembly in 1993, and the *Platform for Action* from the UN Fourth World Conference on Women in Beijing in 1995, are critical international policies that specifically address gender-based violence. They recognise it as a violation of women's and children's human rights, and "as a form of discrimination that prevents them from participating fully in society and fulfilling their potential as human beings."[10] These, and other conventions such as the *Convention on the Elimination of all forms of Discrimination Against Women* (CEDAW) and the *Convention on the Rights of the Child* (CRC),[11] must continue to be used at local, national, and international levels to frame all efforts to eliminate the commercial sexual exploitation of children, because they seek to address the wider structures that condone and perpetuate gender-based violence.

Supply and demand

Socio-economic forces influence both the supply of and demand for sex with children, otherwise known as the "push" and "pull" factors. Vast resources have been invested in recent years into research relating

to the "supply" side, and into initiatives addressing root causes of children's vulnerability to commercial sexual exploitation. While this chapter cannot address the scope of these issues in great detail, it is important to consider in general terms some critical factors "pushing" children into exploitative situations. Commonly recognised factors include:

- poverty
- social dislocation
- family breakdown
- prior experiences of sexual victimisation
- homelessness
- ignorance
- consumer and peer pressure

and

- cultural traditions

Clearly a considerable amount of overlap exists between each of these broad categories, and substantial documentation of the interplay between the "push" factors can be found elsewhere.[12] It is sufficient to state that these factors must be considered in relation to one another in developing a comprehensive policy and programmatic response.

What is essential to this discussion is that every effort must be taken "to criminalise the commercial sexual exploitation of children in all its forms and in accordance with the relevant international instruments, *while not criminalising or penalising the child victims*."[13] Indeed, there must be a shift away from criminalising children that have been victimized, to taking firm legal action against those who create a demand for sex with children, and addressing much more seriously the various factors that lead adults to perpetrate such horrific offences. Again, it is important to keep in mind the underlying element of gender-based violence as we seek to understand the profile of those who sexually exploit children.

Two basic categories of adults who commercially sexually exploit children are those considered to be "situational offenders," and those considered "preferential offenders." A situational offender is someone who does not have a sexual preference for or predisposition to have sex with children. A preferential offender, on the other hand, is someone who has a specific sexual preference for sex with children.[14]

Situational offenders can be classified as either "sexually indiscriminate"[15] or "morally indiscriminate," but both groups typically engage in the criminal activity of sex with children without necessarily feeling any real sexual attraction towards them.[16] Situational offenders may be more prevalent in a transient tourist population than preferential offenders,[17] and tend to be the hardest to identify and prosecute as they typically lead "normal" lives, maintaining relationships with their wives or girlfriends, children and friends.[18] What is most important to recognise in the context of this paper is that "*the criminal activity of situational abusers can only be mitigated by the law*; such men cannot be 'treated'; the only response to their crime is punishment."[19]

Preferential offenders are typically attracted to a specific age and gender of children, and are more likely to prefer boy victims rather than girls.[20] There are conflicting opinions regarding whether this group of offenders is evenly represented across the economic spectrum or is more commonly represented by one socio-economic group, so further research in this specific area would be helpful. Paedophiles fit within the category of preferential offenders, as they "are sexually attracted to children below the age of puberty – in clinical definitions, they are considered to be sexual deviants who target children under the age of 13. Their behavioural patterns are well documented and these patterns can therefore be recognised and intercepted."[21]

Very little reliable data exists concerning the efficacy of psychological treatment and legal punishment of preferential offenders. Much more research is necessary with regard to developing effective methods for reducing rates of recidivism (repeat abuse) – which, in conjunction with increased efforts to identify and intercept potential offenders before they exploit children, are critical in reducing the vulnerability of children to abuse.

Much more information exists about the specific characteristics of situational and preferential offenders, but it lies well beyond the scope of this paper. Suffice to say that the approach of identifying and responding to offenders and their actions, must be specifically tailored to the category of offender. Indeed, "grouping together preferential abusers and situational abusers under-plays the possibility that a man who has otherwise normal relations with adult women might also be abusing minors."[22] At the same time, one basic commonality is found between these two categories of offenders: "a disregard for the identify of the child as a person. To them a child is a commodity, a means to an end, something to be used."[23]

While men have typically represented (and remain) the vast majority of those who commit commercial sexual offences against children, recent studies and cases have shown that women are increasingly involved both as child sex tourists, and as "accomplices" in the recruitment, procuring, and pimping of children.[24]

International legal context

In attempting to tackle the commercial sexual exploitation of children through legal means, it must be recognised that there are both national and international legal mechanisms in place regarding this type of offence.

International law can be defined as:

> The legal principles governing the relationships between nations; more modernly, the law of international relations, embracing not only nations but also such participants as international organisations, multi-national corporations, non-governmental organisations, and even individuals (such as those who invoke their human rights or commit war crimes). – Also termed "public international law"; "law of nations"; "law of nature and nations"; "*jus gentium*"; "*jus gentium publicum*"; "*jus inter gentes*"; "foreign-relations law"; "interstate law"; "law between states" (the word "state" in the latter two phrases is the same as nation or country).[25]

With regard to international law, the treaties most relevant to the commercial sexual exploitation of children include the *Optional Protocol to the Convention on the Rights of the Child* (CRC) *on the Sale of Children, Child Prostitution and Child Pornography* (2000); International Labour Organisation (ILO) *Convention 182 Concerning the Prohibition and Immediate Action for the Elimination of the Worst Forms of Child Labour* (1998); and a *Protocol to Prevent, Suppress and Punish Trafficking in Persons, especially Women and Children*, supplementing the *UN Convention against Transnational Organised Crime* (2000).[26]

Because the commercial sexual exploitation of children is intrinsically linked with the trafficking of women and of children,[27] all three areas require further attention with regard to gathering and utilising data that is disaggregated by age and sex. In research documenting the coercion of women into prostitution, for example, it has been common practice to report figures on ages between 16 and 24, without regard for the fact that those falling within the age bracket of 16–17 years are still considered children under the CRC.[28] Thus, the scope of the impact of commercial sexual exploitation on girls is masked by indiscriminate or undifferentiated data. This means that it will continue to prove extremely difficult to deal with the problems specific to the distinct areas of trafficking of women, trafficking of children, and the commercial sexual exploitation of children. Moreover,

> ...in the case of adults, the human rights approach – the recognition of the right to make informed decisions and choices, even if this includes the choice to remain in exploitative situations – will continue to be an issue of debate and has to be considered in program intervention. In the case of children, the international consensus is to withdraw them from exploitation without delay. Action to combat the trafficking of children can and should be part of action to combat the trafficking of adults.[29]

Another key international legal tool that must be considered in more detail is Article 34 of the CRC:

> State Parties undertake to protect the child from

all forms of sexual exploitation and sexual abuse. For these purposes, State Parties shall, in particular, take all appropriate national, bilateral, and multilateral measures to prevent:

- the inducement or coercion of a child to engage in any unlawful sexual activity
- the exploitative use of children in prostitution or other unlawful sexual practices
- the exploitative use of children in pornographic performances and materials.

Implications of this Convention in regard to the responsibilities of State Parties will be discussed further in the following paragraphs relating to national laws. One last point concerning international law is to note that, in addition to these key policies, in 1990 the United Nations mandated the appointment of a Special Rapporteur of the Commission on Human Rights on the Sale of Children, Child Prostitution and Child Pornography to examine, monitor, and report on these forms of human rights violation.[30]

National law – which can be defined as "the set of rules or principles dealing with specific areas of a given legal system"[31] – can also provide useful mechanisms within the international legal system with regard to prosecution of those who commit commercial sexual offences against children. Each state party to (each nation that has ratified) the CRC is required to set in place appropriate laws and social services in order to prevent such abuse.[32] Where there are gaps in a certain country's legislation or implementation, or where such laws do not even exist, some states have developed extra-territorial legislation to prosecute their own nationals who commit offences abroad, the rationale being "that child-sex offenders should not escape justice simply because they are in a position to return to their home country."[33] Currently, a total of 32 countries have adopted extra-territorial legislation (see Annex).

In addition to the aforementioned international legal instruments, on 17 July 1998, the statute outlining the creation of the International Criminal Court (ICC) was adopted at an international conference in Rome. The Rome Statute, as it is known, allows for the prosecution of individuals for genocide, war crimes, crimes against humanity, and crimes of aggression; moreover, "among the many offences included within the scope of war crimes and crimes against humanity are rape, sexual slavery and enforced prostitution."[34] Provisions within the Rome Statute protect the "safety, physical and psychological well-being, dignity and privacy of victims and witnesses."[35]

In order for the ICC to be put into place, 60 countries needed to ratify the statute. By 11 April 2002, 66 countries had ratified, allowing for the Court to come into full force on 1 July 2002. Jurisdiction of the ICC includes crimes committed by nationals whose governments have ratified the Rome Statute, as well as the territories of those governments.[36] The jurisdiction of the ICC is complementary to that of national jurisdictions, in that it gives the party states "primary responsibility and duty to prosecute the most serious international crimes, while allowing the ICC to step in only as a last resort if the states fail to implement their duty – that is, only if investigations and, if appropriate, prosecutions are not carried out in good faith."[37]

The ICC will indeed provide much-needed international legal enforcement mechanisms to ensure that those who commit crimes, such as the sexual exploitation of children through sexual slavery, will be held accountable. Furthermore, "the ICC will help ensure that these serious crimes, long recognised and abhorred by the international community, no longer go unpunished because of the unwillingness or inability of individual countries to prosecute them."[38]

Another critical tool to support national legislation is the Stockholm *Declaration* and *Agenda for Action*, which was issued in 1995 at the first World Congress Against the Commercial Sexual Exploitation of Children. While not legally binding, the *Agenda for Action* determined to accomplish two major goals by 2000:

- to identify/establish national agendas/plans of action against the commercial sexual exploitation of children

and

- to identify/establish national focal points and collect disaggregated data on the commercial sexual exploitation of children.

All states parties that participated in the first World Congress agreed unanimously and signed onto the *Declaration* and *Agenda for Action*, though since that time many have not fulfilled their commitment to develop their own National Plans of Action. While no specific monitoring mechanisms were put in place, to some extent the UN Special Rapporteur on the Sale of Children, Child Prostitution and Child Pornography, and the Committee on the Rights of the Child were able to assist with monitoring. The international non-governmental organisation ECPAT[39] has played a significant role in monitoring the actions of governments in implementing the Declaration and Agenda for Action, primarily through their publication of annual reviews of progress. There has also been some success in legal reform, and there are indications of increased cooperation and coordination between national law enforcement agencies and Interpol,[40] which is reflected to some extent in the case studies in Section Two.

Why focus on a legislative response?

While elimination of the commercial sexual exploitation of children requires a multi-faceted response, the central importance of a legislative response is that the "law embodies the social contract and can catalyse social change by sending a clear message that violence against women [and children] will not be tolerated."[41] As a member of UNIFEM's Internet Working Group on Violence Against Women pointed out, "The criminal justice system response has clearly played a role in educating the public on what is and is not acceptable in our local community."[42]

A legislative response is absolutely critical, first to end impunity for offenders, and second, to communicate a message to the wider public that commercial sexual exploitation of children will not be tolerated. When national and international laws reflect the reality of those who have been exploited and abused, and when those laws are fully implemented, women and children who have suffered so terribly receive a measure of the justice they deserve and can be better protected from further abuse.[43]

This is not to say that enacting and enforcing laws on the commercial sexual exploitation of children will bring an end to all forms of such abuse. UNIFEM's Internet Working Group to End Violence Against Women argues that

> The effectiveness of legal strategies for preventing and responding to violence should be seen in the context of the status of the rule of law. Absent of the rule of law, strategies for law reform or advocacy in the courts will have limited effect on women's lives. Laws on violence against women will lack legitimacy and the supporting framework of legal and political institutions. In such circumstances, laws cannot be enforced to protect women against violence in a manner consistent with human rights.[44]

While these comments refer specifically to legislative reform regarding violence against women, the same reasoning holds true for other forms of gender-based violence, including crimes relating to the commercial sexual exploitation of children.

Moreover, effective legislative reform is not possible unless it takes into consideration and utilises research and other advocacy tools of organisations working directly with children affected by this exploitation. If, on the other hand, a legislative response is taken in conjunction with broader efforts such as public education, advocacy campaigns, information sharing, and networking, then systems and structures that have condoned and supported gender-based discrimination can be shamed and/or transformed. The following section addresses the specific legal reforms undertaken by five industrialised countries in relation to the commercial sexual exploitation of children.

Section 2: Case studies

This section outlines the history of extra-territorial legislation in five industrialised countries, highlights the strengths and weaknesses of current legislation, and makes note of specific cases associated with implementation of these laws. Canada, the United Kingdom, Australia, the United States of America, and

Germany have been selected as case studies in order to focus on a phenomenon in which children are exploited by those with the capital and freedom to travel abroad, and the power to exploit those who are more vulnerable.

Canada

In May 1997, Bill C-27, *An Act to Amend the Criminal Code*, came into force in Canada. The amendments to Section 7 of the Criminal Code were made to extend the jurisdiction of Canadian courts to include acts of sexual exploitation (both commercial and non-commercial) of children committed by Canadians abroad, including child sex tourism. Section 7 (4.1), (4.2), and (4.3) stipulates that Canadians or permanent residents of Canada could be charged for sexually abusing children[45] through such means as child prostitution, indecent acts, child pornography, and incest, while outside of Canada.[46] The purpose of the legislation was "to deter Canadians from engaging in the sexual exploitation of children in foreign countries, to encourage other countries to enforce their own laws to combat child sex offences, and to provide a means of prosecuting Canadians who have committed child sex offences in other countries but have avoided prosecution in that country."[47]

Bill C-27 also made provisions for special protection of children during their testimony. Section 7 (15.1) provides that a videotape of a child victim's evidence may be admissible even when the child witness no longer remembers all of the details of the offence. Section 486 (2.1) makes provisions for a child to testify from behind a screen or outside the courtroom by using closed circuit television.[48] There are also provisions for a support person to be with child witnesses, under Section 486 (1.2), and for affirming the competency of child witnesses (under the age of 14), under Section 16 of the *Canada Evidence Act*. In addition, the amendments to Bill C-27 and other acts[49] provide for the gathering of evidence and witnesses' testimony outside of Canada through the use of video and audio-link technology.[50]

In 1998, the Criminal Intelligence Service Canada (CISC) initiated a national coordinated law enforcement strategy that focused on child pornography, child prostitution and child sex tourism.[51] Working in partnership with Canadian and international law enforcement agencies, CISC seeks to make the commercial sexual exploitation of children a priority issue within the law enforcement community.[52]

To date, no charges have ever been pursued under the amended Section 7 of the Criminal Code. In March 2001, Bill C-15, also known as the "Omnibus Crime Bill" or the *Criminal Law Amendment Act*, was tabled in the Canadian House of Commons. The Bill proposed new provisions in the Criminal Code that sought to protect children from sexual exploitation involving the Internet, and to strengthen the legislation on non-commercial sexual exploitation by removing the procedural requirement for a formal request from the foreign country in which the crime was committed.[53] At the time of writing, the Bill had not yet come into force.

In addition to federal legislative reform, various initiatives at the provincial level also increased the levels of protection afforded to children from sexual exploitation. Additionally, the Consular Division of the Department of Foreign Affairs and International Trade produced a travel brochure entitled *What No Child Should Endure*, in order to raise travellers' awareness of Canada's legislation on child sex tourism.[54] While over 10,000 copies of the brochure were distributed worldwide, there is cause for concern that there is still a very low level of awareness amongst law enforcement agencies, as there have been no successful prosecutions.

United Kingdom[55]

The UK was one of the last countries in Europe to pass extra-territorial legislation, having justified the delay by arguing that the legislation would be too difficult to implement.[56] The *Sex Offenders Act* was passed in 1997, under substantial pressure from ECPAT International and the Coalition on Child Prostitution and Tourism. This legislation provides for prosecution in the UK of Britons who sexually abuse children while overseas. If convicted, offenders are then listed on the Sex Offender Register.

The first successful conviction under this law was of a 64-year-old campsite owner who abused British

children in France; he was sentenced to three years in prison. This case is unusual in that the assaults were upon British children abroad, and it has been argued that this in fact made a successful prosecution easier as it was less costly and labour-intensive to pursue the investigation than it would have been in a case involving foreign children who lived further abroad.[57]

The main weaknesses of this legislation included:

- Citizens of the UK who have been convicted overseas, and subsequently spent time in prison but then returned to the UK, were not required to register.
- Foreign nationals convicted overseas and who came to the UK were not required to register.
- Convicted offenders did not have to notify the authorities of any intention to leave the UK (now addressed by *The Sex Offenders (Notice Requirements) (Foreign Travel Regulations 2001)*; see below).[58]

The most significant obstacle to prosecution was that the legislation required that the offence be recognised as a crime in both the foreign country and the UK. This double criminality requirement prevented prosecution of offenders if there was no such law in the foreign country concerned. One example of the loophole created is a case in which a British national sexually abused boys in Nepal. The case was dismissed because Nepal did not have similar legislation against sexual abuse of children.[59]

The Association of the Chief of Police Officers in the UK provided a list of other factors making it difficult to investigate and secure convictions for child sex tourism by British nationals:[60]

1. The high cost generated by pursuing extra-territorial prosecutions
2. The fact that it is easier to get convictions on grounds of possession and distribution of child pornography
3. The difficulty associated with tracing children in Third World countries
4. Challenges associated with trying to establish the age of foreign children with any precision
5. The fact that as of January 2000, there had not been any requests for assistance from any governments in South and South-East Asia (areas where there was a high probability that offences might be occurring)
6. All transnational investigations have been lengthy, cumbersome and expensive.

In 2001, *The Sex Offenders (Notice Requirements) (Foreign Travel)* came into force. This regulation was originally a part of a consultation paper, but then entered into force at the end of the consultation period. The main aim of the regulation was to amend the Sex Offender Register, in order that police would be informed of sex offenders from the UK who travelled abroad, allowing them to inform relevant authorities in the country of destination to take precautionary measures to protect children. The regulation also stipulates that UK sex offenders travelling overseas for eight days or more must give notice in person to the police at least 24 hours prior to departing from UK. Giving such notice entails providing police with the date of departure from the UK, specifying the country (or countries) to which the offender is travelling, and stating the point of arrival.

The major weaknesses of *The Sex Offenders (Notice Requirements) (Foreign Travel)* are that offenders:

- only have to give notice if leaving the UK for eight days or more[61]
- are encouraged, but are not legally obliged, to give the police the fullest possible details of their travel plans

and

- only have to register with the police eight days after they return to the UK (yet under the Sex Offender Register, offenders must register within 72 hours).

In July 2001, the Home Office published a consultation paper on the review of Part I of the *1997 Sex Offenders Act*. Its main proposal was to enact an

Order to Register a Sex Offender (ORSO), which would apply to UK and foreign nationals convicted of sex offences overseas who decide to come to the UK. This aimed to close two loopholes in the 1997 Act so that:

- UK nationals convicted overseas and who had spent time in prison overseas would now be required to register upon return to UK, and
- Foreign nationals convicted overseas and who had spent time in prison overseas would now be required to register upon arrival in UK.

Weaknesses of the ORSO include:

- Its method for registration is flawed, in that registration occurs in *ad hoc* manner. Instead of police having to apply to a magistrates' court for an ORSO, offenders should be required to register as soon as they enter the UK.
- the time-consuming process of police having to prove that the person was convicted overseas for a sex offence before being able to obtain an ORSO
- ORSO only applies to convictions on or after 1 September 1997.

Sending "a message of determination"

In June 2001, Mark Towner, a 52-year-old man from Kent, England, was sentenced under the *1997 Sex Offenders Act* to eight years in prison for sexual offences he committed against two Cambodian girls while on a business trip in May 2000. Recent research indicates that British men are among the most frequent abusers of Cambodian children.

Towner was prosecuted for having hired two 7-year old girls for sex, and for having taken photographs of himself having sex with the children and then sending the images to Britain by e-mail.

Judge Warwick McKinnon, in issuing the sentence, told Towner that he was "a danger to young children, and the court must send out a message of determination against people who perform acts on ones so young."

Towner had previously pleaded guilty to 14 charges, including having had sex with a girl under the age of 13.

Source: CNN, "UK Court Jails Man for Cambodian Child Sex," http://www.cnn.com, 18 June 2001, in Nuon Rithy Niron, Yit Viriya and Laurence Gray, *Children's Work, Adult's Play: Child Sex Tourism, the problem in Cambodia*, World Vision International, 2001.

Over the past five years, police authorities have arrested 30 Britons on charges of sexually exploiting children worldwide. Of the 30 charged, three were convicted in the UK for offences in France, Cambodia and the Philippines, and 11 were convicted abroad, including three in the Philippines, two in Cambodia, two in Thailand, one in India, one in Japan, one in Romania, and one in the Czech Republic. One of the men convicted in the UK was Durham Wragg, in January 2001, for child pornography made whilst in the Philippines. Wragg was charged with smuggling, possessing and taking obscene pictures of boys that were then made into films.

Australia

Extra-territorial legislation concerning child sex tourism was first introduced in Australia in 1994, when the Commonwealth Parliament passed the *Crimes (Child Sex Tourism) Amendment Act*. This Act introduced a new "Part IIIA – Child Sex Tourism" into the Crimes Act, covering a broad range of sexual activities committed overseas with children under the age of 16.[62] The Act stipulates that to be held liable,

> ...the offender must have been, at the time of the alleged offence, an Australian citizen or resident; a body corporate incorporated under a law of the Commonwealth, a State, or Territory; or a body corporate that carries on its activities principally in Australia.[63]

While the legislation does not require that the offence be commercial in nature, it does specifically

Critical role of child protection

At the Third Hearing of the International Tribunal for Children's Rights, in Sri Lanka in 1999, Roger Walker of World Vision Myanmar, Naly Piorge of LICADHO and Khou Akha of the Cambodian Centre for the Protection of Children's Rights spoke of a case involving an Australian national who allegedly sexually exploited two Cambodian street children. It took two years to bring the case to court in Australia, where the children were taken to testify against the defendant. The children were apparently subjected to "long periods of aggressive cross-examination in an environment that was alien to them", and "were even unsure about who the defence lawyers were during the committal proceedings". The case ended up being dismissed, the accused was acquitted, and the children were returned to Cambodia having been even further traumatised by the entire process. So while much has already been done to protect children through the enactment of extra-territorial legislation in countries such as Australia, much more must be done to ensure that all actions taken are in the best interests of the child.

Source: *Global Report: International Dimensions of the Sexual Exploitation of Children*[67]

"target those who assist, organise, or benefit from 'child sex tourism'."[64] The legislation makes it an offence to:[65]

- engage in sexual intercourse with a child under 16, while outside of Australia (Crimes Act, s50BA)
- induce a child to engage in sexual intercourse with a third person outside of Australia (Crimes Act, s50BB)
- participate in sexual conduct, such as indecency, involving a child under 16 while outside of Australia (Crimes Act, s50BC)

or

- act or omit to act, whether within Australia or not, with the intention of benefiting from, or encouraging, such an offence; examples include advertising an offer to assist a person to commit an offence (Crimes Act, s50DA and 50DB).

Penalties for committing the aforementioned offences are strict, with imprisonment ranging from 12 to 17 years. It is, however, possible to defend such charges, in cases where:[66]

- the defendant believed at the time of the sexual intercourse or act of indecency that the child was 16 or over (Crimes Act, s50CA); in considering this defence, the jury may consider the reasonableness of the alleged belief (Crimes Act, s50CD)

or

- the child was genuinely married (Crimes Act, s50CD).

The Australian legislation includes a number of strengths worthy of mention. For one, the legislation is fairly comprehensive and has stiff penalties for offenders. It also does not have a double criminality requirement, thus making prosecution possible regardless of whether the country in which the offence was committed actually regards it as an offence. The legislation recognises the evidentiary problems of extra-territorial prosecutions, and thus has provisions for utilising video-link evidence, and allows prosecutions to be successfully pursued without any reference to overseas or child witnesses when sufficient evidence exists within Australia – both of these provisions indicating sensitivity towards child victims and child witnesses.[68] The legislation also contains a forfeiture provision, allowing the government to seize any profits generated by child sex tourism.

The most significant weakness of the *Crimes Amendment Act* is that it only protects children aged 16 or

younger. This falls short of the optimal standard of under 18 set by the CRC.

In regard to implementation of the legislation, the Government has demonstrated positive collaboration with non-governmental organisations (NGOs). In addition to the work of the Australian legislative authorities, NGOs have played a significant role in the formulation, execution, and enforcement of strategies to prevent sex tourism. The media, under pressure from NGOs, has devoted broad coverage to the actions of Australian sex tourists abroad, thereby educating the public on the issue. While the legislation has proven to be effective in prosecuting cases where the offence was committed against children in developing countries, it has also been used successfully in cases of intra-familial sexual abuse of children committed whilst abroad.[69]

One issue of grave concern regarding Australia's capacity to tackle the problem of child sex tourism is that the Federal Government has dissolved the Federal Police Unit responsible for the investigation of crimes relating to child sex tourism, and there are few proactive measures for pursuing sex offenders who travel abroad.[70]

United States of America

In 1994, the US Government passed the *Child Sexual Abuse Prevention Act* (strengthening the Mann Act of 1910), its primary law criminalising child prostitution. The Child Sexual Abuse Act was passed in conjunction with the 1994 *Crime Bill*, and it prohibits interstate commerce for the purposes of prostitution or for any criminal sexual activity. In addition, numerous laws prohibit production, possession, and dissemination of child pornography. For example, the *Child Protection Act* of 1984 specified that all distribution of sexually explicit material involving children was a criminal offence, leading to a substantial increase in federal prosecutions. Despite serious attempts by the Government to protect children in this regard, however, the *Child Online Protection Act, a Communications Decency Act* (1996), and a section of the *Child Sexual Abuse Prevention Act* have "remained largely unenforceable because of civil libertarian claims that they contravene the rights to privacy of individuals."[71]

The Crime Bill, also known as *Act "Title 18 USC Sec. 2423 – Transportation For Illegal Sexual Activity and Related Crimes,"* was passed on 1 September 1994 by the US Congress. The original intent of the Crime Bill was to prevent the transport of women across state lines for sexual purposes. Relating to the sexual exploitation of children, "USC 2423b – Travel With Intent To Engage in Sexual Acts with a Juvenile" reads:

> A person who travels in interstate commerce or conspires to do so, or a United States citizen or an alien admitted for permanent residence in the United States who travels in foreign commerce or conspires to do so, for the purpose of engaging in a sexual act with a person (younger than) 18 years of age that would be in violation of chapter 109A if the sexual act occurred in the special maritime and territorial jurisdiction of the United States, shall be fined under this title, imprisoned for more than 10 years or both.

In essence, the law criminalises travelling to foreign countries for the purpose of engaging in sexual acts with a child (under 18 years of age) if the sexual act would be in violation of US Federal law. The Act has also made it a crime to create pornographic images, and this offence actually carries a stronger penalty than the crime of travelling for the purpose of committing a sexual act.

There are several major weaknesses of the Crime Bill. One such weakness is that it requires that the crime occurred in the course of travel that the offender undertook with *intent* to commit a sexual act. While this is helpful in the prosecution of sex tour operators who package tours for paedophiles or others with the promise of sex with children, it is difficult to establish intent in other types of cases. Legislation is currently pending that would relieve the burden of proving the intent, thus closing this particular loophole.

Another weakness is stipulations within the legislation that it only applies to children under 12 years of age, or children between 12 and 16 years of age. Thus, children aged 16 and 17 are not protected unless the offender uses force, serious threats, or otherwise impairs the victim: "children of this age

are not protected by the new law, particularly in commercial or consensual situations not involving coercion."[72]

No official record has been kept (either by the Government or by NGOs) of the number of prosecutions arising from this legislation, so it is difficult to tell how effective it has been. Moreover, the US Government has not yet ratified the CRC, and has no National Plan of Action for targeting the commercial sexual exploitation of children. However, a landmark case has been brought against a US citizen who operated a child pornography bulletin board system from Mexico to the USA.

Supplementary to the laws outlined above, the USA enacted the *US Victims of Trafficking and Violence Protection Act* in 2000. The intended purposes of the Act include:

- combating the trafficking in persons, which it describes as "a contemporary manifestation of slavery whose victims are predominately women and children"
- ensuring just and effective punishment of traffickers

and

- protecting victims of trafficking.

The Act contains several strong provisions, including:[73]

- a request for US$95 million over two years to support anti-trafficking enforcement and victim assistance programs abroad
- availability of a non-immigrant visa ("T" visa) and protection from criminalisation for trafficking victims in the United States
- a directive that the Secretary of State issue an annual report on the status of international trafficking
- a mandate for establishing an interagency task force on trafficking, and an office at the State Department to monitor and combat trafficking
- doubling of the current penalties for convicted traffickers (up to life imprisonment for worst offences)

and

- a directive that the President deny non-humanitarian aid to countries that tolerate or condone trafficking.

In compiling data and making an assessment of the foreign country, US diplomatic mission personnel are supposed to consult with human rights organisations and other appropriate NGOs. Specified minimum standards for elimination of trafficking, by which foreign countries are assessed, are set out in Section 108, along with actions that will be taken against governments failing to meet these minimum standards, as outlined in Section 110:

> It is the policy of the United States not to provide non-humanitarian, non-trade-related foreign assistance to any government that does not comply with the minimum standards for the elimination of trafficking and is not making significant efforts to bring itself into compliance with such standards.

Section 105 of the Act mandates the formation of an Interagency Task Force to Monitor and Combat Trafficking, to be established by the President of the USA. One key responsibility of this taskforce is to examine the role of the international sex tourism industry in the trafficking of persons and in the sexual exploitation of women and children around the world.

One highlight of this legislation is its strict penalties for offenders. Sex offences committed by force, fraud or coercion, or where the victim is under 14 years of age, range from a fine up to life imprisonment. In all other cases, sentencing ranges from a fine to 20 years imprisonment.

Germany

Under German legislation, a child is defined as a person aged under 14. Under Section 176 of the German Penal Code,[74] those defined as children are guaranteed absolute protection from acts of "en-

gagement in sexual activity with a child or inducement of a child to engage in sexual activity with a third person,"[75] and attempts to commit such acts are also punishable, both with sentences of up to five years imprisonment.[76] A punishment of up to ten years in prison is accorded to those who perpetrate more serious offences involving sexual intercourse, or where the act causes gross abuse to the child.[77] Those between ages 14 and 18 are also afforded certain protections, such that it "is illegal to induce or influence a child under 16 years of age to engage in any sexual activity or to take advantage of their incapacity for sexual self-determination,"[78] and that the age limit for guardians and supervisors is raised to 18 years.[79]

Germany ratified the CRC in 1992, and in so doing, undertook responsibility to protect children from all forms of sexual exploitation. Cases concerning the sexual abuse of children by Germans abroad have been punishable in Germany since 1993, "even if the laws of the foreign country have not been contravened."[80]

Germany reformed its legislation in 1993, and again in 1998, and the Government introduced an *Act to Combat Child Pornography*.[81] Amendments to the German Penal Code in 1998 resulted in further clarification of crimes related to the commercial sexual exploitation of children, in addition to stiffer penalties for such crimes and extension of the statute of limitations for certain serious sexual offences. Procurement of sexual services from minors is prohibited, and Section 180 of the Penal Code stipulates that "anyone who induces or influences a minor to engage in sexual activity for remuneration or for some other reason is liable to punishment."[82] Penalties range from a fine to up to five years incarceration.

While no specific German legislation prohibits child sex tourism, extra-territorial jurisdiction applies, and covers both nationals as well as foreigners.[83] One significant weakness of German legislation is that a general principle of double criminality exists.[84] The only exception is "in cases of sexual abuse of children if the offender is a national and resides in the domestic territory." Another noteworthy point is that "foreigners will only be prosecuted in Germany if a request for extradition from the state where the crime was committed has not been granted or is not possible for any other reason."[85] There have been many extra-territorial prosecutions in recent years in Germany concerning the commercial sexual exploitation of children.[86]

In addition to legislative reform, Germany also issued its National Action Plan (in follow-up to the First World Congress on Sexual Exploitation), and published an addendum to this in 1998, detailing specific issues of commercial sexual exploitation of children that the German Government is seeking to address. Implementation of the National Action Plan and its addendum falls under the responsibility of the Ministry of Families, Seniors, Women and Children.[87] Plans were made to reassess the National Action Plan and its addendum in early 2001.

Comparative analysis of case studies

Such issues as constitutional limitations preventing admissibility of evidence, technological or geographic barriers protecting anonymity of exploiters, and corruption or insensitivity of officials to issues surrounding commercial sexual exploitation undermine global protection of women and children.[88] In the case of countries outlined in this study, none provide full protection to children (under the age of 18) in relation to commercial sexual exploitation, as afforded by the CRC.

The varying levels of success that Australia, Canada, Germany, the UK and the USA have experienced in implementing their various laws is due, in part, to the different measures of cooperation and support undertaken by the tourism industries in each country. For example, in Australia, where an effective and widespread public education campaign targets travellers (in the form of posters and leaflets in airports), police have benefited from higher levels of support from those able to provide tips and evidence for crimes they have witnessed in foreign countries.[89] In the UK, however, where the travel industry is viewed as less supportive of public education, conviction rates are much lower.[90]

Another significant factor affecting differing levels

of success is the degree to which the various governments have been willing to be candid and upfront regarding behaviour of their own nationals abroad. In the UK, government reluctance to acknowledge that UK nationals commit such crimes has delayed legislative reform.

All five countries face similar challenges in regard to

- low levels of reporting
- difficulties obtaining evidence overseas, because of cost, language and cultural differences and locating witnesses, among others[91]

and

- sensitivity and skills required to investigate sexual crimes committed against children.

Section 3: Recommendations

At the Second World Congress Against the Commercial Sexual Exploitation of Children, held in Yokohama in December 2001, a workshop on the topic of extra-territorial legislation highlighted significant lessons learned from implementation. They included "the need for more attention to the evidence of child victims and how it is handled; the need for more awareness-raising among the judiciary, and child sensitive procedures; and the importance of discarding the double criminality provisions in relation to the offenders."[92]

With these lessons in mind, and with the *Yokohama Global Commitment 2001*[93] and the aforementioned comparative analysis in consideration, this report recommends:

1. Enhanced cooperation between legal bodies and NGOs in facilitating prosecution of offenders
    - Experience shows that in most successful prosecutions, police used a combination of official governmental channels and NGOs to obtain evidence.
2. Greater candour and transparency within legislative bodies
    - Unless the highest levels of authority – in place to ensure the full protection of its citizens – can be trusted to act in the best interests of children through open and accountable measures, efforts to protect children from commercial sexual exploitation will prove exceedingly difficult.
3. Better implementation of child-friendly investigative measures and court proceedings
    - Much has been done to develop methods that protect the children from further exploitation throughout investigation and legal proceedings, and that recognise children's right to testify and the value of their testimony. Greater emphasis must now be placed on building the capacity of those involved in facilitating children's participation in legal proceedings.
4. Removal of the double criminality requirement from extra-territorial legislation prohibiting commercial sexual exploitation of children
    - The double criminality requirement has proven to be a significant barrier in facilitation of extra-territorial cases due to weak or non-existent legislation in some countries. The double criminality requirement concerning crimes of commercial sexual exploitation of children must be removed, along with continued emphasis on development of comprehensive domestic legislation for full protection of all children.
5. More collaborative strategies, linking such methods as legislative reform and implementation with public education campaigns
    - The most effective strategies to promote protection of children from commercial sexual exploitation have involved all relevant bodies in developing comprehensive strategies and implementing them through cooperative processes.
6. Developing more democratic processes for participation of civil society – particularly children who have been commercially sexually abused, along with adults who have expertise

Annex: List of countries with extra-territorial legislation

Algeria	Ethiopia	Laos	Slovenia
Australia	Finland	Luxembourg	Spain
Austria	France	Mexico	Sweden
Belgium	Germany	Morocco	Switzerland
Cyprus	Iceland	Netherlands	Taiwan
Canada	Ireland	New Zealand	Thailand
China	Italy	Norway	United Kingdom
Denmark	Japan	Portugal	United States

Source: ECPAT International Survey

in this area – in legal reform, enforcement and monitoring processes

- This includes development of mechanisms by which children can file complaints within their own country or abroad, in addition to appropriate means for children to petition the Committee on the Convention on the Rights of the Child to lodge complaints against state parties.

7. Equipping law enforcement bodies to deal with gender dynamics of commercial sexual exploitation of children and the disproportionately high number of girls that are affected

   - Through gender sensitisation and skills building, law enforcement bodies will be better equipped to respond appropriately to children who have been victimised, as well as to offending parties.

8. Increase coordination and collaboration between law enforcement bodies and psycho-social services, to develop more advanced and effective methods for punishing offenders

   - Recognising the distinct attributes of situational and preferential offenders and responding with the most appropriate methods of punishment is crucial in reducing rates of recidivism.

9. Greater expertise in extra-territorial jurisdiction

   - Heightened awareness amongst law enforcement officers, embassy personnel, NGOs and relevant government ministries of existing legislation and how to implement and enforce it. This expertise is absolutely crucial to ensure effective protection of children.

10. Ongoing commitment to development and implementation of effective national laws and policies (in accordance with the CRC and other relevant instruments and documents) in tandem with a commitment to extra-territorial legislation

    - Whereas extra-territorial law is a crucial tool for elimination of commercial sexual exploitation of children, "it is not a substitute for a trial in the State in which the offence occurred."[94] Both national legislation and extra-territorial legislation must extend full protection to all persons under the age of 18.

Closing

While legal reform and law enforcement are essential tools in the protection of children from commercial sexual exploitation, they must be undergirded with a rich understanding and full recognition of children's rights as human rights.[95] Indeed, protection of children's civil, political, economic, social and cultural rights, and promotion of their full participation in these various spheres, are fundamental to

creating an environment where children are safe from all forms of exploitation. And fundamental to achieving this is the empowerment of boys and girls, along with men and women, in such a way that the rights of all people are respected and nurtured.

Acknowledgement

The author wishes to acknowledge and thank Angela Brouwer for her assistance in the preparation and analysis of the background legal literature for this paper.

References

1 Pino Arlacchi, Executive Director of United Nations Office for Drug Control and Crime Prevention, and UN Under-Secretary General, speaking to government officials at a forum in Sicily on the topic of combating trafficking; referenced in "Mafia Makes Billions from Trafficking People," *Reuters*, 15 December 2000

2 While this report highlights five countries that currently have extra-territorial legislation on child sex tourism, there are 32 states with such legislation. A full list of these is found in the Annex.

3 ECPAT, "Facts and Figures: Even One Child is Too Many," Briefing note to the Second World Congress against the Commercial Sexual Exploitation of Children, 2001

4 M. Cherif Bassiouni, "Sexual Slavery Crosses Moral and National Boundaries," *Chicago Tribune*, 17 February 2002

5 As specified by the UN Convention on the Rights of the Child (CRC). While Article 1 of the CRC definition of a child allows for various interpretations according to national legal systems, by defining a child as "every human being below the age of 18 years unless, under the law applicable to the child, majority is attained earlier," this paper uses the strict term of below the age of 18 years.

6 As specified in *The Yokohama Global Commitment, 2001*, the declaration signed at the closing of the Second World Congress against the Commercial Sexual Exploitation of Children, held in Yokohama, Japan, 17–20 December 2001.

7 http://rhrc.org/resources/gbv/bib/intr.html#a

8 http://mirror.ippf.org/resource/refugeehealth/manual/4.htm#The

9 Geraldine Van Bueren, "Child Sexual Exploitation and the Law: A Report on the International Legal Framework and Current National Legislative and Enforcement Responses," a theme paper to the Second World Congress against the Commercial Sexual Exploitation of Children, 2001, p. 3

10 http://www.unifem.undp.org/trustfund/

11 The Convention on the Elimination of all forms of Discrimination Against Women (CEDAW), adopted by the UN General Assembly in 1979, and the Convention on the Rights of the Child (CRC), adopted in 1989, are two other essential international policies that define women's and children's rights as human rights. They are discussed more fully in relation to their international legal implications in the following section.

12 For more information, please refer to the NGO Group for the Convention on the Rights of the Child and ECPAT International, "Causes and Contributing Factors," briefing note to the Second World Congress against Commercial Sexual Exploitation of Children, 2001

13 *The Yokohama Global Commitment, 2001* (emphasis in italics added by the author)

14 The National Police of Cambodia, *Understanding and Investigating Child Sexual Exploitation: Trainers Manual*, as referenced in Laurence Gray, "Sexual Exploitation and Violence in Cambodia," in Melanie Gow (ed.), *A Safe World for Children: Ending abuse, violence and exploitation*, World Vision International, Monrovia, California, 2001

15 L. Gray, *loc. cit.*, p. 30

16 NGO Group for the Convention on the Rights of the Child and ECPAT International, "People Who Prey on Children," briefing note to the Second

World Congress against Commercial Sexual Exploitation of Children, 2001

[17] L. Gray, *loc. cit.*, p. 30

[18] "People who prey on children", *loc. cit.*

[19] *ibid.* (emphasis added by the author)

[20] L. Gray, *loc. cit.*, p. 31

[21] *ibid.*

[22] *ibid.*

[23] *ibid.*

[24] NGO Group for the CRC and ECPAT International, "People Who Prey on Children", *op. cit.*

[25] Maya Steinitz, "The Role of International Law in the Struggle against Sex-based and Gender-based Violence against Refugee Women", consultancy report submitted to the International Rescue Committee and to the Reproductive Health for Refugees Consortium, March 2001, as referenced in *Black's Law Dictionary*

[26] NGO Group for the CRC and ECPAT International, "Taking Action: Responses and Gaps", briefing note to the Second World Congress against Commercial Sexual Exploitation of Children

[27] Article 3(a) of the *Protocol to Prevent, Suppress and Punish Trafficking in Persons* defines trafficking as "the recruitment, transportation, transfer, harbouring or receipt of persons, by means of the threat or use of force or other forms of coercion, of abduction, of fraud, of deception, of the abuse of power or of position of vulnerability or of the giving or receiving of payments or benefits to achieve the consent of a person having control over another person, for the purpose of exploitation." There is also specific reference to the trafficking of children, such that the "recruitment, transportation, transfer, harbouring or receipt of a child for the purpose of exploitation shall be considered 'trafficking in persons' even if this does not involve any of the means set forth in [the definition]."

[28] Panudda Boonpala & June Kane, "Trafficking of Children: The Problem and Responses Worldwide", a preliminary version of an ILO-IPEC report on the trafficking of children, for distribution at the Second World Congress against Commercial Sexual Exploitation of Children, 2001

[29] *ibid.*

[30] "Extra-Conventional Mechanisms of the United Nations Commission on Human Rights", http://www.unhchr.ch/html/menu2/2/mechanisms.htm

[31] *ibid.*

[32] To date, 191 countries have ratified the CRC. The only two states not to have ratified are the USA and Somalia.

[33] Fiona David, "Child Sex Tourism", *Trends and Issues in Crime and Criminal Justice (T&I)* series, No. 156, Australian Institute of Criminology, June 2000. http://www.aic.gov.au/publications/tandi/tandi156.html

[34] *Global Report: International Dimensions of the Sexual Exploitation of Children,* Montreal, International Tribunal for Children's Rights, 1999

[35] Article 68 of the Rome Statute, as referenced in *Global Report: International Dimensions of the Sexual Exploitation of Children, loc. cit.*

[36] http://www.hrw.org/campaigns/icc/qna.htm - What crimes

[37] *ibid.*

[38] *ibid.*

[39] ECPAT stands for End Child Prostitution, Pornography And Trafficking. ChildWise is one of ECPAT Australia's projects: http://www.ecpat.org/projects.htm

[40] http://www.ecpat.net/eng/ecpat_inter/projects/monitoring/wc2/briefing_note11.asp

[41] "Women @ Work to End Violence: Voices in Cyberspace", Report of UNIFEM's Internet Working Group to End Violence Against Women, http://www.unifem.undp.org/w@work/w@work2.htm

[42] Quote from a member of UNIFEM's Internet Working Group to End Violence Against Women, *ibid.*

[43] *ibid.*

[44] *ibid.*

[45] Children between the ages of 14 to 18 are not protected from all of these offences.

[46] http://lois.justice.gc.ca/en/1997/16/5277.html#rid-5278

[47] http://www.cisc.gc.ca/AnnualReport2000/Cisc2000/exploit2000.html

[48] http://www.voyage.gc.ca/Consular-e/Publications/child_fact-e.htm

[49] Bill C-40, an Act respecting extradition, to amend the *Canada Evidence Act*, the Criminal Code, the *Immigration Act* and the *Mutual Legal Assistance in Criminal Matters Act*, and to amend and repeal other Acts in consequence

[50] *ibid.*

[51] http://www.cisc.gc.ca/AnnualReport2001/Cisc2001/exploit2001.html

[52] *ibid.*

[53] *ibid.*

[54] ECPAT International, *Five Years After Stockholm: 2000–2001*, Bangkok, 2001, p. 62

[55] The author wishes to acknowledge Heidi Keme, Child Rights Officer, World Vision UK, for her assistance in the research on British legislation concerning the commercial sexual exploitation of children.

[56] Jeremy Seabrook, *No Hiding Place: Child Sex Tourism and the Role of Extraterritorial Legislation,* Zed Books, London, 2000

[57] J. Seabrook, *loc. cit.*, p. 99

[58] Statutory Instrument Number (S.I.) 2001, No. 1846.

[59] *ibid.*, p. 95

[60] *ibid.*, p. 94

[61] ECPAT International is currently campaigning for change in this regard.

[62] F. David, *loc. cit.*

[63] Crimes Act, s50AD, cited in F. David, *loc. cit.*

[64] *ibid.*

[65] *ibid.*

[66] *ibid.*

[67] *Global Report: International dimensions*, 1999, *op. cit.*

[68] *ibid.*

[69] *ibid.*

[70] ECPAT International, *Five Years After Stockholm: 2000–2001*, p. 154

[71] *ibid.*

[72] Margaret A. Healy, "Prosecuting Child Sex Tourists at Home: Do Laws in Sweden, Australia and the United States Safeguard the Rights of Children as Mandated by International Law?", *Fordham International Law Journal*, Vol. 18, May 1995, No. 5

[73] Joseph Mettimano, *Information Brief: Sexual Exploitation of Children*, World Vision US, 2002

[74] http://www.interpol.int/Public/Children/SexualAbuse/NationalLaws/csaGermany.asp

[75] http://www.ecpat.net/eng/Ecpat_inter/projects/monitoring/online_database/countries.asp?arrCountryID=64&CountryProfile=&CSEC=Overview,Prostitution,Pronography,trafficking&Implement=Coordination_cooperation,Prevention, Protection,Recovery,ChildPartic

[76] http://www.interpol.int/Public/Children/SexualAbuse/NationalLaws/csaGermany.asp, *op. cit.*

[77] *ibid.*

[78] http://www.ecpat.net/eng/Ecpat_inter/projects/monitoring/online_database/countries.asp?arrCountryID=64&CountryProfile=&CSEC=Overview,Prostitution,Pornography,trafficking&Implement=Coordination_cooperation,Prevention,Protection,Recovery,ChildParticipation&Nationalplans=&orgWorkCSEC=&DisplayBy=optDisplayCountry, *op. cit.*

[79] *ibid.*

[80] http://www.child-hood.org/en/home_p445.html

[81] http://www.ecpat.net/eng/Ecpat_inter/projects/monitoring/online_database/countries.asp?arrCountryID=64&CountryProfile =&CSEC=Overview,Prostitution,Pronography, trafficking &Implement=Coordination_ cooperation, Prevention,Protection,Recovery,ChildParticipation &Nationalplans=&org WorkCSEC=&DisplayBy=optDisplayCountry, *op. cit.*

[82] *ibid.*

[83] *ibid.*

[84] *ibid.*

[85] *ibid.*

[86] *ibid.*

[87] *ibid.*

[88] Canadian Component of the Protection Project, 1 July 2000

[89] J. Seabrook, *loc. cit.*, p. 95

[90] *ibid.*

[91] *ibid.*

[92] Vitit Muntabhorn, "Report of the Second World Congress against Commercial Sexual Exploitation of Children", loc. *cit.*, p. 25

[93] *The Yokohama Global Commitment 2001* is the document signed by the governments that participated in the Second World Congress Against the Commercial Sexual Exploitation of Children, reaffirming the commitments that were made at the First World Congress and pledging further action.

[94] Van Bueren, *loc. cit.*, p. 16

[95] *ibid.*, p. 12

Finding a way forward: Gender-based violence in Tanzania

Ruth Kahurananga and Monalisa Kileo

Introduction

Tanzania has been progressing towards gender equality, especially after making national commitments following the 1995 Fourth World Conference on Women in Beijing.[1] Multi-party, democratic elections have taken place, and civil society – notably non-governmental organisations (NGOs) – has energetically addressed gender issues. However, on the gender-related development index (GDI) of the United Nations Development Programme (UNDP), Tanzania ranks number 140 out of 162 countries.[2]

The African and UN Charters on Human Rights clearly indicate that violence against women and girls (or gender-based violence) is a violation of human rights globally.[3] In Tanzania, as well as other African countries, patriarchal culture or male-dominated ideologies have justified oppressive gender relations; for example, wife battery is considered culturally acceptable, by some men as well as women, as a form of discipline.

Violence against women includes any act, omission or conduct in which physical, sexual or mental suffering is inflicted directly or indirectly.[4] This can be through deceit, seduction, harassment, coercion or any other means. Its aim is to intimidate, punish or humiliate the woman or girl. This in turn undermines women's sense of security, leads to lack of self-confidence and diminishes physical or mental capacities.

According to newspaper reports in Tanzania, violence against women has increased at household levels, work, schools and public places.[5] It is now considered to include many no longer-tolerated behaviours such as female genital mutilation (FGM), wife battery, rape, child molestation, violence against elderly women (such as those subject to allegations of being witches), sexual exploitation, and abuse of household domestic workers ("house girls").

This paper primarily concentrates on domestic violence, FGM, and violence against elderly women. Types and extent of domestic violence in Tanzania are discussed, illustrated by statistical data from the Tanzania Media Women's Association (TAMWA). The paper then considers the phenomenon of violence against elderly women, mostly in relation to allegations of witchcraft, which is prevalent in the Shinyanga, Mwanza and Tabora Regions of northwestern Tanzania. The harmful traditional practice of FGM is then examined, in terms of its short- and long-term effects, myths and facts surrounding the practice, and the challenges to its eradication.

It is argued that in seeking to combat these types of violence against women in Tanzania, various issues need to be addressed, such as women's legal capacity, gender imbalances in decision-making, unequal opportunities in education and employment, as well as existing policies. Finally, this paper suggests a way forward and recommendations, including advocacy by civil society groups, political empowerment of women, and gender budget initiatives.

Types of violence against women and girls

The most common manifestations of violence against women are physical, sexual, psychological and economic abuse. Physical violence means harmful attack on the body, whereas psychological, emotional or mental violence can be manifested in confinement, deprivation of financial and personal resources as well as in verbal abuse.[6]

Gender violence can be understood to include physical, sexual and psychological harm occurring especially in families. Figure 1 shows the different dimensions of domestic violence, with the primary cause of violence, namely power and control exercised by men over women, in the centre. These can be in the

form of battering, restrictions on movement, sexual abuse of female children in households, economic abuse, dowry-related violence, marital rape, or FGM and other harmful traditional practices. The age range of victims as reported in Southern Africa Development Community (SADC) countries was from six months to 50 years old.[7] The social construction of gender roles places women as property and dependents of male "protectors", making women vulnerable to violent treatment by men.

Reasons given for women's deaths due to violence

The Ministry of Home Affairs prepared a report on the statistical data available on violence against women. The study documented a total of 1,551 deaths in the period from January 1996 to September 1998 (Table 1).

- In the four cases of death due to cattle rustling, three of the women were owners whereas one woman died during the theft. This would be found mainly in pastoral communities where one clan or tribe raids and plunders another's cattle.
- Regarding the deaths due to robbery, 31 of the women were the property owners whereas two died in the process of committing the crime.
- With 500 victims, witch-hunts of elderly women were the second leading cause of death.
- Domestic violence was divided into two groups, namely violence in local bars (ugomvi vialbuni) and violence at home (ugomvi majumbani). Both domestic violence and adultery could be combined together as causes of death, since the latter is often used as a reason to inflict violence against women. Together, domestic violence and adultery/jealousy took 557 of 1,551 lives, making it the leading cause of violent deaths to women.
- Women with mental disabilities died either from causing bodily harm to themselves or being attacked by other mentally disabled people.
- "Other reasons" included death in which the cause was not officially known.

Power and control by men of spouse/partner through violence

Physical Violence: Push, grab, beat and/or burn; use of weapons; rape and murder

Sexual Violence: Coerce to engage in sexual activity; treat as sex object; physically attack sex organs

Reproductive Control: Deny access to contraceptives; forced sterilisation

Using Children: Use children to relay messages to induce guilt and to harass

Threats and Intimidation: Make and/or carry out threats to harm emotionally or physically, including threats of abandonment, poverty, suicide, physical violence or murder.

Economic control: Unfair control of household income and assets; prevent spouse from obtaining or keeping a job; take money and other possessions

Isolation: Control who spouse sees, talks to and goes; Seclude from friends and family

Emotional abuse: Insult; demean; play "mind games"

Source: Sisterhood Is Global Institute, 1998[8]

Domestic violence: wife battery and abuse

In Tanzania, most men pay dowry for their wives. In some cases, men view their wives as their property or asset; something they bought. This attitude gives rise to marital problems from battery to killings of wives.[9] According to 1997 reports from TAMWA, between 1990 and 1995 there were 2,022 cases or wife beating, reported and recorded. Table 2 lists the number of reported cases of different types of violence against women in Tanzania.

Table 1: Reasons and number of deaths of women
from January 1996 to September 1998 [10]

Cause of death	1996	1997	1998	Total
Cattle rustling	2	1	1	4
Robbery	2	23	8	33
Witch-hunt of elderly women	170	194	136	500
Theft	–	14	1	15
Domestic violence	127	95	110	332
Adultery/jealousy	72	69	84	225
Accidental death	13	6	9	28
Revenge	12	6	0	18
Women with mental disability	2	3	–	5
Other reasons	137	149	105	391
Total	537	560	454	1,551

Source: TAMWA, *Sauti ya Siti*, 1999

Wife battery or abuse is a common practice among the Wakurya tribe in Mara region. This act has injured and humiliated many women, and in extreme cases, led to death. As expressed by 35-year-old Nyangeta Amos: "Men beat us because they are the ones in authority. We are the wretched ones." [11]

As reported by the Serengeti District Commissioner, Colonel Labani Makunenge, to TAMWA staff, wife battery is a traditional way of life among the Wakurya. Acceptance of this means, unfortunately, that most women do not report battery. In addition, women fear greater retaliation, and that they would humiliate their parents, if they reported it – the dowry can be as high as 40 cattle, and few parents would be willing to return this amount to the son-in-law should their daughter leave him. For these reasons, many women living in abusive relationships adopt a culture of silence.

Some tribes are considered to be more violent than others. Yet even among the most educated citizens, spousal battery occurs. Previously, this and other forms of domestic violence were mainly reported in the regions along Lakes Victoria and Tanganyika, the northern regions of Kilimanjaro and Arusha, as well as the central regions such as Dodoma. The major cause for this brutality was cited as alcoholism. For instance, in an interview with TAMWA, the Acting Dodoma Regional Police Commander, Masele Urasa, stated that most murders occurred during the harvest season when community members, es-

Table 2: Reported cases of wife beating, rape, violence against elderly women, and child sexual abuse

Type	1990	1991	1992	1993	1994	1995	Sub-total
Wife-beating	357	292	295	420	451	207	2,022
Rape	94	111	144	864	702	517	2,432
Violence against elderly women	77	82	96	92	120	54	521
Child sexual abuse	81	77	65	365	127	111	826
TOTAL	**609**	**562**	**600**	**1,741**	**1,400**	**889**	**5,801**

Source: TAMWA Files, 1997 found in Nkhoma-Wamunza et al., 1998

pecially men, engaged in excessive drinking. Also during the traditional dance ceremonies, there are many accusations of adultery causing jealousy, resulting in wife battery.[12] A lawyer with the Tanzania Police Force College in Dar-es-Salaam, Abdulrahman Kaniki, concluded that alcoholism and jealousy were the two main causes of wife battery in the Lake Victoria regions in 1996.

Discussions held with Judge Pelagia Khadai of the High Court, Dodoma Zone,[13] revealed that in the Tanzanian cultural setting, most women are not eager to report spousal abuse. Some women believe it is one of the burdens of marriage and should be accepted. Women also stay in abusive relationships either because they would have no custody of the children or they cannot inherit any of the family's property. Obstacles that abused women encounter are:

- inaccessible and unaffordable legal assistance
- insufficient inheritance, and
- fear of violent retaliation by the husband or relative, even leading to death.

The following court cases tried by the High Court, Dodoma Zone, indicate that alcoholism, jealousy and women's subordination perpetuate domestic violence leading to death.

Witch-hunts of elderly women

Among most ethnic groups within Tanzania, elderly people have historically been respected, given authority and viewed as having wisdom. The extended family cared for elderly women and men, providing them with shelter, food, clothing and health care. In most rural communities this is still the case.

Nevertheless, with the introduction of Western culture, greater emphasis is placed on a market economy, the nuclear family, privatisation of the service sector and materialism.[14] This has negatively affected the social fabric associated with caring for the elderly. In some ethnic groups, specifically the Sukuma in Shinyanga, old women are accused of being witches and killed. This practice is also prevalent in Mwanza and Tabora regions, especially in cases with old women who have reddish eyes (due to cooking over smoky firewood), an affliction perceived as a bad omen. These women are harassed, ostracised from their communities, molested, brutally beaten and frequently killed, often being burned alive. In 1994 there were 3,693 deaths due to allegations of witchcraft in Tanzania, and 60% of these cases were women.[15]

These killings were orchestrated by the community. The strong cultural belief in witchcraft in these communities within Shinyanga and Mwanza perpetuates this practice. For instance, a person might consult a

Examples of domestic violence cases leading to homicide reported and tried by the High Court, Dodoma Zone, in 2001

Case 1 – Dodoma District Court, 1999

The accused (husband) directed the deceased (wife) to sell two kilograms of sugar. Unfortunately, the deceased used an empty tin container to measure the sugar instead of the measuring scales. A quarrel ensued, the accused hitting the deceased with a stick and piece of pipe on the head. The accused was convicted of manslaughter on 1 February 2001.

Case 2 – Dodoma District Court, 1999

On 3 April 1997 the deceased (wife) and accused (husband) went to their neighbours' house to drink local brew, pombe. On their way home the deceased went to collect fuel-wood while the accused proceeded home. The deceased returned home after it was dark, and because of this was kicked by the accused in her abdomen as well as her head. She died of rupture of the spleen with extensive internal haemorrhage and brain damage. The accused was convicted of manslaughter on 7 May 2001.

Case 3 – Mpwapwa District Court, 1999

The parties (husband and wife) suspected one another of having extra-marital affairs. On the day of the incident, the accused (husband) claimed that he heard his wife (deceased) making plans to meet another man. When the accused came home, he stabbed his wife five times. He was convicted of manslaughter on 19 March 2001.

Case 4 – Singida District Court, 2000

The killing occurred on 22 September 1998 at Mtama Village, Singida. The deceased (wife) and accused (husband) returned home late and were both drunk. Upon arrival, the accused demanded that the deceased prepare a meal, but the latter declined. A misunderstanding occurred between the two, followed by a fight. During the skirmish, the accused struck the deceased with a stick and kicked her abdomen. The deceased died of head injury. The accused was convicted of manslaughter on 22 September 2001.[16]

traditional healer for a range of reasons. The traditional healer has herbs and other natural medicinal products that can be used to cure physical ailments, and performs divination either to explain a client's future or to identify why the client has a 'curse.' In the case of the latter, the traditional healer may vaguely suggest that there is an old woman or man who is bewitched and is the one causing all the misfortune. The primary suspects tend to be old women who live alone, but who are surviving relatively comfortably; people believe that these old women are doing so well because they are bewitched. Once the client has deduced who the "culprit" is, they may hire contract killers within the community who are secretly known. The old women are usually hacked to death using machetes.

Some of the deaths can be attributed to greed. Traditional healers earn income from these consultations, and in some cases they will continue divination whether they believe their counsel is true or false. Moreover, when elderly women have property like a large farm (*shamba*), their relatives, neighbours or community members may covet this, and accuse the elderly women of being witches in order to obtain these assets.[17] These false accusations, clearly driven by greed, can lead to fear and mob violence where these women lose their property as well as their lives.

In 1928, the colonial government enacted the *Witchcraft Ordinance* as criminal law. However, analysis revealed that rarely were witch-hunters arrested.[18] Several reasons were given as to why this was the case:

- Murders were committed at night, making it difficult to identify the killers.
- Killings were considered family secrets since no one wanted to admit that one of their family members was considered to be a witch.
- If any information about a killing was shared, this was seen as being sympathetic to or in collaboration with the "witch."
- Witch killings were orchestrated by hired groups known to the community; sometimes these killers were brazen enough to tattoo the corpse with their mark as a form of advertising their services.[19]
- Some of the areas where the murders occurred were extremely remote and not easily accessible by law enforcers.
- Even the traditional law enforcer known as the *Sungusungu* may have either advocated or participated in the killings; one of the essential qualities of a *Sungusungu* was to be able to identify witches within the community.
- The opinion of some community members is that government officials are not keen to report witch killings for fear that they will become unpopular with the community, and be ousted from power through local elections.

The Tanzanian elite, including law enforcers, perceive that killing old women is a problem of rural people who are uneducated heathens. Clearly, any solutions to stop these murders will have to come from within the community itself.

Female genital mutilation (FGM)

In the international community, female genital mutilation (FGM) is seen as a violation of the human rights of women and girls. The tendency to assert one's own culture in opposition to human rights, no longer holds, and human rights have been given supremacy over any other set of values. More recently, international human rights documents have begun to specifically identify FGM as a human rights issue.[20]

Tanzania has signed and ratified the Convention on the Rights of the Child (CRC) following the 1990 World Summit on Children, as well as the following Conventions:[21]

- *Convention on the Elimination of all forms of Discrimination Against Women* (CEDAW), 1979, ratified in 1984
- The *African Charter on the Rights and Welfare of the Child*, 1990
- The Beijing Platform for Action, 1995

Tanzania's Parliament also passed the *Sexual Offences Special Provisions Act* of 1998[22] which states in section 21 that:

> Any person with the care, control and custody of a girl child under 18 years of age who causes that girl child to be genitally mutilated is guilty of an offence and liable to imprisonment for a term not less than 5 years and/or a fine.

Furthermore, the *Penal Code* of 1981,[23] in section 169A states that:

> It is an offence to assault anyone and genitally mutilate a person over the age of 18 without their consent.

FGM is a tradition or cultural practice that involves total or partial removal of the outer parts of the female genitalia.[24] WHO reported four types of FGM classified by the World Health Organization (WHO) globally, namely:[25]

- **Type 1**: partial or total removal of the clitoris (this practice is known as *clitoridectomy*)
- **Type 2**: removal of the clitoris and all the parts of the labia minora (known as *excision*)
- **Type 3**: cutting away all external genitalia and stitching of the two sides of the vulva, sealing parts of the urethra and vagina, only leaving a small opening to allow for the passage of urine and menstrual blood (known as *infibulation*)

Table 3: Cultural beliefs and myths *vs.* facts about FGM

Cultural beliefs and myths	Facts
It is necessary to perform FGM as part of the initiation ceremony and informal training as a rite of passage from being a girl to becoming a woman.	The growth of a girl and the training in moral ethics are important rites of passage, not mutilating female organs.
After the FGM ceremony, a girl becomes eligible to get married.	These days men prefer to marry girls who have not undergone FGM.
Women and girls who have been mutilated are more culturally accepted and respected in their community.	Women and girls who are educated and engaged in developing their community are worthy of acceptance and respect.
FGM is a method of reducing women's libido, so it does not exceed that of men.	A woman has equal rights as men to have pleasure during the sexual act.
FGM reduces promiscuity and adultery.	Adultery and promiscuity is a behavioural practice and not reduced or stopped by performing FGM. There is no difference in the prevalence of adultery between the women who are mutilated and those who are not.
The gynaecological disease known as *lawalawa*, which causes vaginal itching, is cured by FGM.	Proper hygiene, cleanliness and antibiotics are crucial for avoiding gynaecological diseases.
FGM improves fertility.	FGM causes infertility.
It is said that FGM is a tradition.	Harmful traditional practices and customs should be discontinued.
FGM facilitates easy and safe delivery.	A woman's life is endangered during delivery if she has undergone FGM.
It is believed that FGM enables women to enjoy intercourse more.	Women who undergo FGM experience severe pain, not pleasure, during intercourse.

Source: Kilimanjaro Inter-Africa Committee (KIAC)

- **Type 4**: all types of operations done on the female genitalia such as piercing or excising of the clitoris and/or labia; stretching of the clitoris and/or labia; cauterisation, scrapping or cutting certain parts of the vagina; and introduction of corrosive materials in the vagina.

In a baseline survey conducted by World Vision Tanzania,[26] the first two types of FGM were practised in Dodoma and Arusha regions. In Tanzania, approximately 3 million (10%) of women and girls undergo FGM, mainly in Arusha, Dodoma, Kilimanjaro, Singida and Mara regions. Other regions have a smaller percentage of the population practising FGM, chiefly in Morogoro, Iringa, Lindi and Mtwara.

Myths and facts about FGM

Understanding why FGM is practised enables programmers, planners and activists to develop strate-

gies for its elimination. In Table 3, a copy of a poster printed by the Kilimanjaro Inter-Africa Committee (KIAC), the first column outlines reasons why most communities practise FGM based on their cultural beliefs, while the second column counters the myths. Using posters like this helps raise awareness and hopefully brings behaviour change in communities that practise FGM.

Short-term effects of FGM

1. The practice is extremely painful and no anaesthesia is given. It is a brutal act indicating lack of pity and care on the part of the ones selected to implement the practice. After prohibition of FGM by the Government, through the *Sexual Offences Special Provisions Act*, the practice has gone underground and in most cases under unhygienic conditions.

2. Usually, damage is caused to the urethra since most of the excisors are very old and some have poor eyesight.

3. There is loss of a large amount of blood, which may cause dizziness, fainting and sometimes death.

4. The unhygienic conditions and unsterilised instruments used for FGM are sources of many infectious diseases such as tetanus and HIV/AIDS and other sexually transmitted diseases (STDs). The wound can become gangrenous leading to death.

5. Other effects include stress and shock which may cause trauma, fainting and even death.

Long-term effects of FGM

6. The damage caused to the urethra due to the excisors' lack of precision or poor eyesight may block or reduce the size of the urethra after healing. Also, the painfulness of the wound makes the girl retain urine for the first few days after mutilation, since urination becomes painful; urine retention leads to formation of uric acid in the bladder, which causes bladder infections and damage to urinary organs.

7. Psychological complications occur such as fear, anger, bitterness, mood instability, nightmares and sleeplessness.

8. Painful sexual intercourse may lead to reduction or loss of sexual pleasure. As a result there are strained marital relations possibly resulting in men becoming unfaithful – thereby increasing the woman's risk of contracting STDs, including HIV/AIDS.

9. One of the results of undergoing FGM is the formation of vaginal scars that are not elastic enough to allow for the passage of a baby during birth. Labour is then prolonged, leaving the baby and mother exhausted after delivery and sometimes causing death.

10. Inelasticity of the vagina causes FGM victims to rupture or require incision during delivery, to allow sufficient space for the baby to pass. This leads to excessive bleeding during delivery, sometimes even death.

11. Vaginal infections caused by unhygienic instruments may spread throughout the reproductive tract leading to infertility.

Successes and challenges in eliminating violence against women in Tanzania

The Government, NGOs and communities have had some success in reducing violence against women in Tanzania. However, there are still factors that perpetuate it. The successes and challenges are due to patriarchal ideology and socialisation; legal capacity; poverty; gender disparities; access to opportunities in education, training and employment; accountability and responsibility of government ministries; and policies.

Culture, socialisation, patriarchal ideology

Culture is the totality of people's ways of life, values, beliefs, social practices and ideology.[27] Clearly, culture may be a source of liberation or oppression. The extended family is one positive cultural practice that should be maintained. Another is the traditional credit system known as *Upatu*, formed by

women's groups or networks, which acts as a revolving fund and enables members of a group to support one another especially during times of economic crisis.

Patriarchal ideology means a social system where men are dominant and women subordinate; the former having power, ownership and control over resources such as land, the latter being powerless and having few or no ownership rights.[28] In such systems, men are considered to have more social worth and superiority compared to women. These behaviours, attitudes and practices are perpetuated as girls and women are socialised with these negative stereotypes both in the family setting and culturally. Boys learn that their social value is greater since they are permanent members of the family; meanwhile, girls are viewed as a commodity with which dowry can be earned. They will leave their families to join their husbands, so they have no ownership rights either in their parental homes or their new homes. FGM and witch-hunts of old women are culturally rooted in socialisation and patriarchal ideology.

Legal capacity

In Tanzania there is a multiplicity of laws (customary, religious and statutory) that deal with marriage, inheritance and custody of children. These often lead to discrimination against women, in spite of constitutional provisions on equality of all women, men, girls and boys.[29] Although there have been several efforts to sensitise women and men on these laws, most women are unaware of their basic rights. In addition, the legal system is overburdened with cases, but lacks resources like staff and funds; therefore the utilisation of statutory laws is slow and cumbersome.

NGOs such as TAMWA, the Tanzania Gender Network Program (TGNP) and Tanzania Women Lawyer's Association (TAWLA) have made immense strides in raising awareness on women's rights and disseminating information on the constitutional laws. Others like the Women's Legal Aid Centre (WLAC) and the Legal and Human Rights Centre (LHRC) have provided legal aid to women in different regions of the country.

Within the Tanzanian Government, there is an economic wing known as *Shirika la Kutetea Wanawake Tanzania* (SUWATA) that also started a legal clinic to counsel women legally and defend them in court.[30] SUWATA handles cases dealing with marriage, inheritance, custody and maintenance of children, and employment contracts.[31] Through weekly legal aid clinics, many women have been assisted. Sometimes, if the man is the cause of the violence, he may be counselled as well. Fortunately, several cases have been resolved out of court.

Through the *Sexual Offences Special Provisions Act* of 1998, the Government has shown commitment to combating violence against women. Organisations like World Vision Tanzania, TGNP and the Kilimanjaro and Dodoma Inter-Africa Committees (KIAC and DIAC) have advocated for the elimination of harmful cultural practices like FGM and early marriage, and have promoted girl child education.

Poverty among women

Micro-enterprise development (MED) has achieved enormous success in addressing poverty among women. For example, the Small Enterprise Development Agency (SEDA), a parallel organisation of World Vision Tanzania, has managed to raise the living standards of women in various towns. Other MED organisations have flourished with considerable success. Poverty reduction is the main national development goal that is supported by activities of the Government, NGOs and the rural community.

The gap between rich and poor is widening, especially between the urban and rural populations. This leads to rural women carrying more of the workload – even though traditionally they have no property rights – so in cases of domestic violence, these same women have neither a place to flee to nor a means of making a living. Even where credit facilities are available women may have access but no control over their money and other resources. When new technology is introduced into a community, especially if it will generate income, men take it over whereas the women continue with low skills, knowledge and productivity.

Gender disparities in decision-making

There have been steps taken, albeit some controversial, by the Government to enhance women's participation in decision-making.Through affirmative action, 25% of village and district councils should be women.There have also been initiatives to increase women's participation in village committees on critical issues such as water and sanitation management.[32] One of the Government's post-Beijing commitments was to increase women's political empowerment.

In Tanzania, women do not influence the decision-making process either at domestic or national levels.[33] At the household level, for instance in the allocation of domestic resources, existing attitudes of the patriarchal society view men as the decision-makers, and women as being voiceless. At the national level, few women are appointed to high-profile positions, thus limiting their influence in management, planning and the decision-making process within the country.

Opportunities for education, training and employment

Unequal secondary and tertiary education continues to hinder the advancement of women and girls. The education curriculum is stereotyped and does not encourage girls and women towards careers leading to positions of influence.This is also due to the socialisation of girls and women, which sets predetermined sex roles. Mathematics, technical and science subjects are geared towards boys since they are socialised to be more career oriented. Table 4 illustrates the considerable differences in school enrolment for females and males, starting in Form 5. After graduating from secondary school, there is also a sharp drop of female students in technical training and university.

Pregnancy and absenteeism also hinder girls from completing their education. Existing societal attitudes favour the promotion of boys' education at the expense of the girls'. Access to employment opportunities is also unequal for women and men.

Accountability and responsibility of government ministries

The Ministry of Community Development, Women Affairs and Children (MCDWC) in Tanzania mainland and the Ministry of State, Women and Children Affairs (MSWC) in Zanzibar are responsible in coordinating, monitoring and facilitating the concerns of women in the state. These Ministries also have an advocacy role in mainstreaming women and gender issues in the other Ministries and sectors. In 1987, gender focal points were appointed in all Ministries and they were mandated to interact with established women in development/gender and development (WID/GAD) units in NGOs and international organisations in order to mainstream women and gender issues. However, this strategy was not very effective due to the following reasons:

- Both MCDWC and MSWC lacked an institutional mechanism in terms of capacity and organisational structure to coordinate, facilitate and monitor gender mainstreaming.
- With the exception of the Civil Service Department, which established a gender unit,

Table 4: Enrolment in educational institutions, 1994

Educational Level	Girls/ Women (%)	Boys/ Men (%)
Primary Standard I	49.2	50.8
Primary Standard 7	49.4	50.6
Secondary Form I	45.8	54.2
Secondary Form 4	43.4	56.6
Secondary Form 5	31.6	68.4
Secondary Form 6	27.1	72.9
Teacher education training	50.8	49.2
Technical education	6.0	94.0
University education	21.8	78.2

Source: Bureau of Educational Statistics of Tanzania.[34]

other Ministries only appointed gender focal points. Furthermore, the gender focal points were not situated in positions of influence.

- It is not mandatory for Ministries, institutions or sectors to plan, implement, monitor and evaluate their work with a gender perspective.

Policies

A policy is a crucial instrument in realising development objectives since it gives direction on a common understanding. In Tanzania, development plans are based on a general national policy, however there are specific sectoral policies. These include the *Child Development Policy* (MCDWC, 1996), *Education and Training Policy* (Ministry of Education and Culture, 1995), *Community Development Policy* (MCDWC, 1996), and the *Women in Development and Gender Policy* (MCDWC, 2000). Specific WID/GAD policies and inclusion of women's issues in sectoral policies is one of the efforts made by the Tanzanian Government to mainstream gender issues. However, the analysis done by the Sub-Programme for Women's and Gender Advancement revealed the following problems:

- Implementing gender mainstreaming has been a major drawback despite the fact that the WID and GAD policies of the United Republic of Tanzania include advocacy for women and gender mainstreaming.
- Furthermore, WID policies have not clearly defined and distinguished the difference between WID and GAD. As stated by the Sub-Programme for women's advancement,

  > While a focus on women is recognised as legitimate in its own right, GAD has emerged to be a much more effective policy approach providing a clear conceptual rationale for planning to meet gender needs of both women and men for sustainable development.[35]

- Data separated by gender are lacking in several sectors so it is difficult to analyse the impact of the various policies on women and men separately.

The current policies in Tanzania are in three categories:

- The first category has a general perspective. The policies on Agriculture and Energy are examples.
- The second category encompasses those with a WID perspective, treating women as special, marginalised groups. Policies of employment, population, education, trade and industry fall in this category.
- The third category of policies emphasise a welfare approach that focuses on improving women's reproductive roles and to a lesser extent their productive roles. These include population and land policies.

A way forward and recommendations for combating violence against women in Tanzania

From the early 1990s Tanzania experienced political reform that brought about a multi-party democracy. This, in turn, led to different forms of independent media and created opportunities for the active participation of civil society.[36] Specifically in the realm of gender, various activists have developed an informed civil society, with activities ranging from lobbying and advocating to networking and coalition building. Advocacy and lobbying by coalitions and networks in civil society can bring about change. In the 1990s, various initiatives ensured that issues of violence against women were brought to public attention and legal redress demanded.

Recommendations for addressing domestic violence

Some issues that aggravate wife battery and abuse are patriarchal ideology, economic recession or hardships, and increased indebtedness at the household level.[37] The *Declaration by Heads of State or Government of the Southern African Development Community and the Prevention and Eradication of Violence Against Women and Children*,[38] of which Tanzania is a signatory, succinctly outlines key recommendations for eliminating violence against women. The solution is

enforcement and implementation of the SADC recommendations.

1. Passing laws such as sexual offences and domestic violence legislation stipulating that violence against women is criminal, with appropriate measures of penalties, punishment and enforcement is crucial.
   - Fortunately in Tanzania there is the *Sexual Offences Act*, 1998. More work needs to be done in disseminating information about this Act as well as CEDAW.
2. Protecting and empowering women, girls and elderly women through appropriate measures is necessary.
3. There is a need for eliminating gender biases so that justice and fairness is shown to both the victim and accused.
4. Effective access to counselling, restitution and reparation for women and children subjected to violence. Some examples of this are the Counselling Centre operated by TAMWA as well as the Women's Legal Aid Centres found in various regions.
5. Adopting strategies to prevent and eliminate violence against women and girls are crucial.
6. Eradicating harmful traditional practices, stereotypes and religious beliefs that legitimise and exacerbate violence against women and girls is important.
   - As shown in this paper, FGM falls under this category.
7. Introducing and supporting gender sensitisation and public awareness programmes will help eradicate violence against women.
8. Ensuring that the media appropriately educates the public on the adverse effects of violence against women and girls as well as the discontinuation of negative stereotypes.
9. Providing accessible, affordable and effective services such as information, responsive police, legal services or legal aid, social welfare to women and children.
10. Promoting gender sensitisation and training for all service providers such as the judicial officers, prosecutors, police, prison, welfare and health officials.
    - In Tanzania, most of the key public officials are men occupying decision-making positions. In the civil service women comprise 19% of senior to middle management; 12% of the police force and 3–4 % as heads of departments and units; and 5–7% of primary and district court magistrates.[39]
11. Researching and documenting information on violence against women and children – specifically, the causes, prevalence and consequences – is important.
12. Sharing best practices and experiences on eliminating violence against women and children at all levels, namely national, regional and international.
13. Ensuring that integrated implementation by all stakeholders occurs.
14. Allocating essential resources to ensure implementation, monitoring and sustainability.

Recommendations for addressing witch-hunts of elderly women

A study carried out by the Government in 1992 provided some useful recommendations in addressing the practice of witch-hunting elderly women. These included improving literacy levels, technology for productive and domestic activities, and also the economic condition of both women and men.[40] However, little has been accomplished to date. NGOs' efforts to address the problem have also been minimal, although NGOs have concentrated more on women's economic empowerment.

In the past, elderly people were looked after by their children and relatives. Three possible reasons why this traditional familial care has decreased are:

- The unemployment rate has increased so people have greater economic hardships.

- The moral obligation for caring for the elderly has been weakened in the communities. In urban areas, for instance, the high cost of living does not socially or economically promote the extended family structure.
- Thirdly, HIV/AIDS has put additional stress on most households who use their limited resources in caring for the sick.

What is needed is the establishment of efficient mechanisms for collective accountability to the elderly. Social security schemes need to be established in both rural and urban settings. There are approximately 44 institutions for the elderly and destitute, 20 being run by the Government.[41] In urban locations, there are some institutions such as "Getting Old is to Grow" (GOIG) that must be extended to the rural areas. However, culturally, most old people are not used to being isolated and confined in homes for the aged, and there have been incidences where old people have preferred to be destitute in their own community than to live in institutions. A preferable system would be community-based care, which has been shown to be effective especially in looking after people in the advanced stages of HIV/AIDS.

Budget and cost implications cannot be ignored. Unfortunately, when budgets are being allocated, gender sensitivity is not addressed. It is important to have gender-disaggregated data to adequately address the needs of men and women, girls and boys. If budgeted for, services such as social security funds, saving schemes and community-based aged care would be able to assist elderly women accused of being witches and chased from their communities.

Recommendations for combating FGM

Advocating for FGM eradication initiatives need to change the attitudes of community members to this harmful traditional practice.[42] This can be achieved through educational campaigns aimed at policy makers, influential members of the community, as well as children – especially the girl child and her parents. The following recommendations have been made by World Vision Tanzania through its extensive work in reducing FGM:

- Prevention and eradication of such practices should be based on education about their adverse health-related, psychological and socio-economic effects.
- Target groups such as civil society staff, community leaders, religious authorities, health professionals, traditional birth attendants, mutilators, parents, schoolchildren, teachers, women, youth groups and men need to be involved.
- Managers should be trained to facilitate change in stereotypes, beliefs and attitudes towards gender issues among field staff and communities.
- Production of information, education and communication (IEC) materials is necessary to enhance efforts for public and government advocacy.
- In order to influence a change in attitude towards the practice of FGM, the use of advocacy tools may be the most effective method as it entails the use of influential members of the community.
- Involving all members of the community in the advocacy initiative ensures ownership and the possibility for lasting change.

Activities such as community and national mobilisation, education campaigns, production of publications, child participation, training of trainers are crucial. For the mutilators themselves, alternative means of earning an income need to be addressed.

The following true story illustrates the complexity of FGM issues:

Naitovuaki's story

Naitovuaki* was born on 18 March 1985 in a Masai community in Simamjiro District, Tanzania. In 2001 she completed Standard Seven (primary education) and received a pass mark of 55% from Olbili Primary School.

A few months ago her life was turned up-

side down. Her father wanted her to undergo FGM so that she could become eligible for marriage in the near future. However, Naitovuaki knew that this was a painful ceremony both physically and emotionally. Through the grassroots advocacy work being done by World Vision in her community, she gained knowledge and awareness of the harmful effects of FGM as well as the importance of child rights and responsibilities. Fortunately she had an ally who opposed FGM – namely her grandmother, who was literate and had received some basic education. Her grandmother advised the mutilator not to mutilate Naitovuaki and her sister, even though they went through the initiation ceremony, which lasted for days. So they feigned immense pain so that their plan would not be discovered.

Soon after the FGM ceremony, Naitovuaki's father decided that she would marry a rich elderly man who practised polygamy; she would be his fifth wife. Naitovuaki wanted to continue her education, but the minimum grade to enter a government secondary school was 62%. She was not eager to marry this old man, so she asked her uncle to enable her to run away from home. Naitovuaki realised that her right to education was being violated. Her uncle took her to the World Vision Area Development Program, where Naitovuaki stayed with the project coordinator, who later brought her to the Advocacy Unit of World Vision Tanzania. In collaboration with the Regional Social Welfare Office (RSWO), the Women's Legal Aid Centre (WLAC) and the Human Rights Centre (HRC) in Arusha, World Vision Tanzania started addressing the issue. The RSWO wrote a letter to her father in order to establish dialogue and counsel him.

According to Tanzania's *Marriage Act*, 1978, a girl cannot be married under the age of 15 but after that she may be married with parental consent. This contradicts the *Convention of the Rights of the Child* (CRC) and the *African Charter for the Rights and Welfare of the Child*, which states that a child (under the age of 18) should not be married, and Tanzania has ratified both the CRC and the African Charter.

The RSWO and the NGOs involved in the case agreed that Naitovuaki should be facilitated to leave her home environment and further her education. With initial funding from World Vision, she was enrolled at Emusoi Sisters' Centre that has assisted several Masai girls in the same predicament to start pre–Form One (secondary) education. At the end of the academic year, if her grades improve she will be sent to a secondary school for the next four years.

Unfortunately, the situation at home continues to be rocky, as Naitovuaki's mother has been sent away by her father. The father also threatened to discontinue the education of the rest of his children, citing Naitovuaki as a bad example.

* Recorded January 2002. Real name withheld to protect her identity

Closing

Gender-based violence takes many forms in different countries. This paper has reviewed three forms prevalent in Tanzania. However, there are variations in levels and types of violence across different regions within the country. For instance, in Arusha Region FGM is prevalent, but it is not practised in Kagera Region.

Advocating for the eradication of violence against women needs to result in proper enforcement of existing laws, policies and conventions, as well as implementation of policies through strategic programming. For instance the *Sexual Offences Special Provisions Act* of 1998 clearly defines those acts punishable by law such as FGM and violence.

The Government, NGOs, individuals and community-based organisations (CBOs) have managed to network and work together to advocate for change; this should continue. The Government can hold civil society accountable, and vice versa.

When a belief is deeply rooted in culture, such as FGM and the witch-hunting of elderly women, it is even more essential to raise awareness of its adverse effects through publications, media and informational, educational and communications material. Positive cultural practices can be celebrated as a way of combating oppressive ones.

References

[1] B. Keller & D. Kitunga, *Towards Gender Equality in Tanzania, A Profile on Gender Relations,* Tanzania Gender Networking Programme (TGNP), Swedish International Development Cooperation Agency Secretariat for Policy and Socio-Economic Analysis, Stockholm, 1999, pp. 8, 9, 30–32

[2] The GDI adjusts the average achievement of each country in life expectancy, educational attainment and income in accordance with the disparity in achievement between men and women. UNDP, *Human Development Report*, Oxford University Press, New York, 2001, pp. 210–213

[3] United Republic of Tanzania, *Tanzania Women, Part I, Women in Mainland Tanzania*, Country Report to the UN Fourth World Conference on Women, Beijing, China, September 1985, Government Printer, Dar-es-Salaam, 1995, pp. 10–19

[4] M. Mhoja, & H. Kijo-Bisimba, "Tanzanian Customary Laws of Inheritance: A Case Study of Cultural Violence Against Women" in *Women Challenging Violence, Experiences from Eastern and Southern Africa*, Friedrich Ebert Stiftung, Dar-es-Salaam, 1994, pp. 2–8

[5] A. G. Nkhoma-Wamunza, K. Katalyeba, P. Mayeye & A. Mwasha, *The Rights of Women and Girls in Tanzania: A Study on Knowledge, Attitudes and Practices with a Gender Perspective in Twelve Selected Districts*, A Study Report Initiated and Sponsored by UNICEF, UNICEF, Dar-es-Salaam, 1998, pp. 82–102

[6] A. Abate & F. Phiri, eds, *A Training Manual on Gender in Food Security for Planners and Managers*, Food Security Training Project, Harare Zimbabwe and University of Namibia, Windhoek, undated, pp. 70–74

[7] Abate & Phiri, *ibid.*

[8] Sisterhood Is Global Institute, *Safe and Secure: Eliminating Violence Against Women and Girls in Muslim Societies*, Montreal, 1998.

[9] TAMWA, *Sauti ya Siti, ibid.*

[10] Tanzania Media Women's Association (TAMWA), (Chama Cha Wandishi Wa habari Wanawake Tanzania (CHAWAHATA)), *Sauti ya Siti*, A Tanzanian Women's Magazine, 15 December – 15 January 1999, pp. 8, 16–17, 21

[11] *ibid.*

[12] ibid.

[13] Judge Pelagia Khadai, High Court Dodoma Zone, private discussions, Dodoma, 2001

[14] F. Mukangara & B. Koda, *Beyond Inequalities: Women in Tanzania*, Tanzania Gender Networking Programme, Women in Development Southern Africa Awareness, and Southern African Research and Documentation Centre, Dar-es-Salaam & Harare, 1997, pp. 56–59

[15] Mukangara & Koda, *ibid.*

[16] *Random Data Collection Irrespective of Cause of Death in Homicide Matters*, High Court Dodoma Zone, 2001

[17] Nkhoma-Wamunza et al., *ibid.*

[18] J. Mihangwa, *Violence Against the Aged: The Case of Killings on Witchcraft Beliefs in Shinyanga Region*, Tanzania Media Women's Association, Dar-es-Salaam, 2000, pp. 41–43

[19] Mihangwa, *ibid.*

[20] Advocacy Unit, World Vision Tanzania, *Advocating for FGM Eradication in Tanzania*, Proposal submitted to the Civil Society Challenge Fund, World Vision UK and Department for International Development (DfID), Arusha, 2001, pp. 19–22.

[21] United Republic of Tanzania & UNICEF, *The Way Forward with Children and Women*, Government

Printer, Dar-es-Salaam, undated, p. 19

[22] United Republic of Tanzania, *Sexual Offences Special Provision Act*, Acts Supplement to the *Gazette of the United Republic of Tanzania*, No. 27, Vol. 79. Government Printer, Dar-es-Salaam, 1998

[23] United Republic of Tanzania, *Penal Code*, Chapter 16 of the Laws (Revised), Principal Legislation, Issued Under Cap. 1, s. 18, Government Printer, Dar-es-Salaam, 1981

[24] Advocacy Unit, World Vision Tanzania, *Female Genital Mutilation (FGM): Baseline Survey Report in Central and Arusha Zones*, Arusha, 2000, pp. 8–12

[25] WHO Fact Sheet, Female Genital Mutilation, April 1997

[26] Advocacy Unit, World Vision Tanzania, 2000, *Op.cit.*

[27] United Republic of Tanzania, *Tanzania Women, Part 1: Women in mainland Tanzania*, Country report to the UN Fourth World Conference on Women, Beijing, September 1985, Dar-es-Salaam, Government Printer, 1995, pp. 10 – 19

[28] Keller & Kitunga, *op. cit.*

[29] Southern African Development Community (SADC), *Sub-Programme for Women's and Gender Advancement, 1997/98–2003*, Associated Printers, Gaborone, 1998, pp. 53–57

[30] United Republic of Tanzania, 1995, *op. cit.*

[31] Mhoja & Kijo-Bisimba, *op. cit.*

[32] Keller & Kitunga, *op. cit.*

[33] Southern African Development Community (SADC), *Sub-Programme*, *op. cit.*

[34] Bureau of Educational Statistics, Tanzania, Adapted from a presentation in *Towards Gender Equality in Tanzania*, Tanzania Gender Networking Programme (TGNP) & Southern African Research and Documentation Centre (SARDC), Associated Printers, Gaborone, 1997, p. 43

[35] Southern African Development Community (SADC), *Sub-Programme*, *op. cit.*

[36] Keller & Kitunga, *op. cit.*

[37] Mukangara & Koda, *op. cit.*

[38] Southern African Development Community (SADC), *Gender and Development: A Declaration by Heads of State or Government of the Southern African Development Community on the Prevention and Eradication of Violence Against Women and Children*, Addendum to the 1997 *Declaration on Gender and Development* by SADC Heads of State or Government, Associated Printers, Gaborone, 1998, pp. 20–24

[39] Keller & Kitunga, *op. cit.*

[40] Mukangara & Koda, *op. cit.*

[41] *ibid.*

[42] Advocacy Unit, World Vision Tanzania, 2001, *Op.cit.*

Rape as genocide: Lessons from the Balkans and Rwanda in the 1990s

Brenda Fitzpatrick

Introduction

> "It's war," he shrugged. "Rape happens."[1]

> "I think the reticence [of international courts to try cases of rape] is a combination of classic gender discrimination, that manifests itself in the attitude that crimes of sexual violence against women are so-called lesser crimes."[2]

Rape was established as a form of torture and of cruel and inhumane treatment and, as such, a war crime, by the Geneva Conventions of 1949.[3] But the decade of the 1990s saw heightened awareness of rape as a weapon of war rather than a more limited notion of it as a by-product of unruly troops engaged in conflict.

Rape was widespread in the conflicts in the Balkans and in Rwanda in the 1990s. An Ecumenical Women's Team from the World Council of Churches, visiting refugee camps in and around Zagreb in 1992, reported: "Survivors speak of 'rape on the front line' and 'third-party rape'. These are rapes carried out publicly by Serbian soldiers to demoralise family members and opposition forces compelled to witness them."[4] In 1993, the United Nations Economic and Social Council (ECOSOC) in a human rights resolution expressed outrage at rape being used as a weapon of war[5] and in 1994, the UN General Assembly's resolution 205 expressed alarm at "the continuing use of rape as a weapon of war."[6] Both of these resolutions also recognised the use of rape as an instrument of ethnic cleansing and noted that "the abhorrent policy of ethnic cleansing is a form of genocide" – thus a definite link was made between rape and genocide.

If the Balkans and Rwanda conflicts were genocides, the question needs to be asked: Were the rapes, which were part of the conflicts, 'genocidal'? or were they 'accompanying violations of rights'? In either case, they were horrendous acts and there can be no hierarchy in the respective definitions. However, it is as important to understand the nature of rape and genocide, as to understand the nature of killing and genocide, if the international community is to have any chance of prohibiting, preventing, recognising, responding to, prosecuting and punishing these practices.

The Genocide Convention

Key elements of the text of the 1948 *Convention on the Prevention and Punishment of the Crime of Genocide*[7] (the Convention) are issues of defining and identifying the perpetrators, the targeted victims, the nature of the acts, the intent behind those acts and the responsibility to prosecute. There have been many criticisms of the Convention: some have criticised it for being too limited in scope[8] and others for being unenforceable.[9] Yet, even taken in its current minimalist form, it is a useful way of analysing and understanding events that demand attention – events which include mass rapes.

Within the terms of the Convention, it would seem that the rapes in the 1990s in Rwanda and in the Balkans (especially in Bosnia-Herzegovina), could be deemed genocidal in that they were potent elements of genocidal campaigns. In each arena, it is possible to identify perpetrators and targeted victims; there is an established responsibility for prosecution; and the nature of the rape fits within the definition of the Convention. In each case, intent to destroy "in part or in whole," especially as it causes "serious bodily or mental harm to members of the group" can be established.[10]

The International Criminal Tribunal for Rwanda (ICTR) ruled that rape and sexual violence "constitute genocide in the same way as any other act as long as they were committed with the specific in-

tent to destroy, in whole or in part, a particular group targeted as such."[11] In Rwanda, rapes, which were most often the precursor to killing, were part of one integrated genocidal campaign. In the Balkans, where many rapes targeted women who were then left alive, rape would seem to have been a parallel campaign in which rape on its own could be defined as genocidal.

That numerous and extensive acts of rape occurred in both arenas is well documented.

The Balkans

By December 1994, in the former Yugoslavia, there were approximately 1,100 reported cases of rape and sexual assault. About 800 victims had been named or were known to the submitting source; about 1,800 victims had been specifically referred to but not named or identified sufficiently by the reporting witness; and witness reports through approximations referred to a possible further 10,000 victims.[12] The European Council received a report from an Investigative Mission in January 1993 which accepted the possibility of speaking "in terms of many thousands. Estimates vary widely, ranging from 10,000 to as many as 60,000. The most reasoned estimates suggested to the Mission place the number of victims at around 20,000."[13]

These numbers and the limited mandate of the Mission (to investigate only treatment of Bosniak women) were later criticised,[14] though such criticisms were offset by the acknowledged reluctance of many women to report rapes. The report of the Commission of Experts[15] outlines some reasons for this reluctance. They included fear of reprisals against themselves and family members; shame and fear of being ostracised; as time passed, many women just wanted to get on with their lives; for many women did not have a place to report the assaults or rapes; and increased scepticism by refugees about the international community's response.

Reports by Human Rights Watch including *Bosnia and Hercegovina, "A Closed Dark Place": Past and Present Human Rights Abuses in Foca*,[16] and by writers such as Peter Maas, detail many individual incidents.[17]

Rwanda

Human Rights Watch has published an extensive documentation of events in Rwanda and claims that "at least half a million people perished" in the thirteen weeks after April 6 1994.[18] Throughout the 771 pages of this documentation there are constant references to rape of women although there is no attempt to quantify it. In the publication *Shattered Lives,* Binaifer Nowrojee says, "Rwandan women were subjected to sexual violence on a massive scale" and "Although the exact number of women raped will never be known, testimonies from survivors confirm that rape was extremely widespread and that thousands of women were individually raped, gang-raped, raped with objects such as sharpened sticks or gun barrels, held in sexual slavery (either collectively or through forced "marriage") or sexually mutilated."[19] Reasons for Rwandan women not always reporting rape are noted as similar to those of women in the Balkans.

I was in the refugee camps at Ngara, Tanzania, during the massive exodus from Rwanda in 1994. These camps were filled with refugees who were surviving Tutsis and some Hutus who had been targeted in the massacres. A prevailing belief of the aid workers and medical and relief personnel was that any Tutsi "female" (this term was often used to include both women and little girls of any age) who had managed to cross the border to safety had "probably been raped – and maybe more than once."[20] Tutsis were targeted "because of their Tutsi origin and not because they were RPF [Rwandan Patriotic Front] fighters. In any case, the women and children would, naturally, not have been among the fighters."[21]

Before considering the issue of policy-related rape, it is essential to consider whether rape *per se* can fall within Article II of the Convention – that is, to determine whether rape is an act that can be committed "with intent to destroy, in whole or in part" a targeted group:

Genocide Convention, Article II

In the present Convention, genocide means any of the following acts committed with intent to destroy, in whole or in part, a national, ethnical, racial or religious group, as such:

(a) Killing members of the group;

(b) Causing serious bodily or mental harm to members of the group;

(c) Deliberately inflicting on the group conditions of life calculated to bring about its physical destruction in whole or in part;

(d) Imposing measures intended to prevent births within the group;

(e) Forcibly transferring children of the group to another group.

According to Helen Fein, Raphael Lemkin – the 20th century activist scholar who coined the word 'genocide' – viewed (b), (c) and (d) above as steps towards (a) in most cases of genocide. Fein also notes: "besides mass killing, genocide also may include...murder through starvation and poisoning of air, water or food and...the involuntary transfer of children."[22] Rape is a notable omission from her list, considering that rape can contribute to mass killing and that it can also be shown to cause serious bodily or mental harm, to deliberately inflict conditions of life calculated to bring about physical destruction, and to impose measures intended to prevent births within the group.

"In whole or in part": rape's destruction

Many women in Rwanda were killed after being raped, but some did survive. Rwanda is a country where HIV/AIDS has been rampant since before 1994. Nowrojee noted the persistent health problems of surviving victims of sexual abuse during the genocide and, "According to Rwandan doctors, the most common problem they have encountered among raped women who have sought medical treatment has been sexually transmitted diseases, including HIV/AIDS (although it is often impossible to know if this is due to the rape). Since abortion is illegal in Rwanda, doctors have also treated women with serious complications resulting from self-induced or clandestine abortions arising from rape-related pregnancies." There have also been health problems arising from pregnancies and childbirth among extremely young girls who were raped. This is compounded by the fact that "the stigma surrounding sexual abuse often dissuades women from seeking the medical assistance they need."

Many women are rejected by communities – or suffer feelings of guilt for having survived after rape. In one case reported from the Balkans by Human Rights Watch, a woman taken from her family and husband and returned an hour later, fainted and wept. "She told her mother-in-law and other women in her family that she had been raped. In shock, she tried to commit suicide by putting her fingers in a light socket." In another interview a woman is quoted: "I am afraid I am pregnant. If it's true that I am pregnant, I'd rather die."[23] Reports from Rwanda include reference to some women who, after being raped, were told they would be allowed to live so that they would "die of sadness."[24] A Rwandan colleague now living in London told me the story of her cousin, a mother before she was held by *Interahamwe* soldiers, frequently raped and eventually allowed to escape. "We still worry about her. She will not leave her house now and for a long time she did not care for her child. They did it to humiliate her and they destroyed all her ability to live."

The group impact of rape is described by Nowrojee: "The humiliation, pain and terror inflicted by the rapist is meant to degrade not just the individual woman but also to strip the humanity from the larger group of which she is a part. The rape of one person is translated into an assault upon the community through the emphasis placed in every culture on women's sexual virtue: the shame of the rape humiliates the family and all those associated with the survivor."[25] Additional to this is the long-term impact on a group when many of its women suffer physical and psychological injuries, and possibly encounter economic difficulties when deprived of traditional support of husbands and community who may ostracise victims or blame or suspect them of complicity with the enemy.[26]

Children of rape

Other deaths have resulted from children being abandoned or from infanticide. The Rwandan National Population Office estimated between two and five thousand pregnancies resulting from rapes. These

are referred to as "pregnancies of the war," "children of hate," "*enfants non-desirés* (unwanted children)" or "*enfants mauvais souvenirs* (children of bad memories)."[27] In 1992, I was in the former Yugoslavia speaking with doctors and health workers with Bosnian refugees who had crossed into camps near Zagreb. Many of these workers spoke of women who were raped and who had either committed suicide or killed children born of the rapes.

Article II refers to "measures taken to prevent births," but follows this with the words "within the group." In patriarchal societies such as Rwanda and the former Yugoslavia, however, children are recognised as belonging to the group of the father. In the Bosnian refugee camps, it was stated to me that children whose biological fathers were Serbs would always be considered in some way Serb. The speaker, a professional woman, continued, "One part of me – deep inside – believes that my children belong to their father."[28] Not only are the children of the rapes seldom accepted as not part of the mother's ethnic group, they are also often the cause of family divisions when mothers try to raise them.

There are clear grounds for admitting rape as a potentially genocidal act according to Article II of the Convention.

There are also clear grounds for establishing 'intent to destroy' with rape in both the Balkans and in Rwanda.

Rape as opportunism, rape as policy

While there are accounts of rape by all sides in both the Balkans and in Rwanda, the evidence is that most were committed against Bosniak women by the Serbian forces[29] and against Tutsi women by much of the Hutu population and forces of the *Interahamwe* in Rwanda.[30] In its 1998 ruling that Jean-Paul Akayesu, a former mayor, was guilty of genocide, the ICTR included rape in the genocidal acts. In the summary of the case against Akayesu, one Tutsi woman is recorded as testifying: "each time that you met assailants, they raped you."[31] These statements and the corroborating evidence presented to the court would seem to offer an alternative view to that reflected in Stoett's comment that, "Even the Rwandan massacre can be interpreted as largely political."[32] In both arenas, there are clear indications of acts targeting "a national, ethnical, racial or religious group, as such,"[33] thus meeting the Convention's criteria for genocide.

However, it is important to note the different types of rape reported in both arenas. The ICTR Summary noted that at that time (2 September 1998) there was "no commonly accepted definition of this term in international law," and went on to offer a definition of rape as "a physical invasion of a sexual nature, committed on a person under circumstances which are coercive," noting that, "in this context, coercive circumstances need not be evidenced by a show of physical force."[34] Bassiouni identifies several different categories of rape, which included that committed as the result of individual or small group conduct "without evidence of command direction or an overall policy," and urges a distinction "between 'opportunistic' crimes and the use of rape and sexual assault as a method of 'ethnic cleansing'." The two types of rape that can be identified as related to ethnic cleansing are those occurring as part of a policy of commission, and those that point to a policy of omission.[35]

Fein has said that "one can demonstrate intent by showing a pattern of purposeful action," and referred to Reisman and Norchi who argued that intent "is demonstrated on *prima facie* grounds by deliberate or repeated (criminal) acts."[36] The patterns, which emerged in accounts of rape in Bosnia, have been well documented.

Bassioni's report to the UN Security Council identified recurring characteristics of rapes and sexual assaults and concluded that, while some cases were the result of independent individual or small group conduct, the patterns suggested that "a systematic rape and sexual assault policy exists." While admitting that this was yet to be proven, he noted that some level of organisation would have been needed to account for the large number that occurred – particularly in places of detention. When considering the correlation between media attention and the decline in the number of rapes and assaults, he sug-

gests, too, "that the purposes for which the alleged rape and sexual assault was carried out had been served by the publicity." This, in turn, "would indicate that commanders could control the alleged perpetrators, leading to the conclusion that there was an overriding policy advocating the use of rape and sexual assault as a method of ethnic cleansing."[37] The rapes documented in the report on Foca by Human Rights Watch[38] indicate a systematic approach. ECOSOC referred to "the systematic practice of rape" being used in the ethnic cleansing,[39] and the General Assembly noted the conviction that "this heinous practice constitutes a deliberate weapon of war in fulfilling the policy of ethnic cleansing."[40]

The conclusion of the World Council of Churches report *Rape of Women in War,* state that there was "mounting evidence of systematic rape." In the same report, a woman representative of a mosque in Zagreb is quoted: "There has been rape in every war – all soldiers raped...but before, it was always a thing of shame."[41] The patterns documented in the texts already mentioned indicate both a deliberate plan of rape and assault, and widespread condoning of these acts – indicating both a policy of commission and a policy of omission.

Later, Kosovar refugees fleeing the Serb forces also reported systematic rape. I was in Albania and interviewed a spokesman for a group of attorneys working with the General Prosecutor of Albania. He believed that there were grounds for international investigation based on the evidence he had been documenting. He spoke of the large numbers of women prepared to testify, despite the reticence he would have expected of victims of rape, and concluded that one reason was "the collective nature and aspect of the crimes. Sadly, when many women have been raped, it may be easier for each one to cope and to speak about her experience."[42]

Similar evidence has emerged for Rwanda. Nowrojee wrote, "The genocidal intent behind sexual violence in the Rwandan genocide emerges from both the overall pattern of sexual violence and the individual cases of abuse documented in different parts of the country during different phases of the genocide. The pattern of sexual violence in Rwanda shows that acts of rape and sexual mutilation were not accessory to the killings, or, for the most part, opportunistic assaults. Rather, according to the actions and statements of the perpetrators, as recalled by survivors, these acts were carried out with the aim of eradicating the Tutsi." Documented cases recall rapists saying during the acts that they wanted to kill all Tutsi (though, as noted above, some told of attackers saying that rather than kill the women on the spot, they preferred to "leave them to die from their grief"). One woman told of her rapist saying, "We must kill Tutsi women. We must rip them apart." Rape was "condoned and encouraged by the army and government authorities" and "the genocide planners deliberately created and permitted a generalised environment of lawlessness."[43]

A further indicator of intent is the evidence of deliberate impregnation of women raped. Bassiouni identified this in the former Yugoslavia. When describing the patterns of rape and sexual assault, he wrote, "Often the captors state that they are trying to impregnate the women; pregnant women are treated better than their non-pregnant counterparts; and pregnant women are detained until it is too late in the pregnancy to obtain an abortion." He identified particular characteristics of rapes and sexual assaults: "perpetrators tell female victims that they will bear children of the perpetrator's ethnicity, that the perpetrators were ordered to rape and sexually assault them" and "perpetrators tell victims that they must become pregnant and hold them in custody until it is too late to get an abortion."[44]

Additional evidence of intent is found in the propaganda that preceded the genocide in Rwanda. Media such as Radio Kangura and RTLM, virulent tools of propaganda, fuelled the hatred and jealousy of Tutsis in Hutu listeners. Tutsi women – traditionally seen as beautiful, desirable and seductive – were presented as spies and enemies of the Hutu. Kangura was reported as warning Hutus "to be on guard against Tutsi women," since the fighters of the RPF "will not hesitate to transform their sisters, wives and mothers into pistols" to conquer Rwanda.[45]

Prunier points out that when identifying the "organisers" of the events in Rwanda, "doubts are rela-

tively limited." Until the late stage "the killers were controlled and directed in their task by civil servants in the central Government," who, in turn, received orders from the capital, Kigali.[46] This is supported by a record dated 6 May 1994 in which prefectural authorities decided to write to burgomasters about the need to stop rapes with violence.[47]

Article II applied

It would seem, then, that the rapes in both Rwanda and in the Balkans can be aligned with Article II of the Genocide Convention. They were perpetrated by identifiable groups, targeted identifiable groups, there is evidence of destruction "in part or in whole of a group as such," and there is clear evidence of intent. Fein[48] has said, "Genocides, states of terror, and states of violation of life integrity often overlap in time in the same place." It is tempting, in acknowledging this, to suggest that the rapes in Rwanda and the Balkans – particularly in Rwanda where so many women were raped before killing – were accompanying violations of rights. However, examination of available reliable evidence must lead to the conclusion that while there were accompanying violations, these acts of rape themselves were genocidal.

Prosecution

Naming a series of acts as genocide brings with it a responsibility to prosecute. This is well recognised by states and the international community. It was for this reason that politicians in Europe and the USA prevaricated for so long before being prepared to refer to events in Rwanda and the Balkans – particularly in Bosnia-Herzegovina – as genocides.

Andreopoulos[49] raised the issues around prosecution referring to Fein's observation that the most fundamental problem with the Convention is "its unenforceability, as the perpetrator of the genocide, the state, is responsible for its prosecution." He has commented that "a transnationalist approach can gather momentum seriously only if it is prepared to tackle the thorny issues associated with the primacy of state sovereignty." Stoett has outlined difficulties in enforcing prosecution given the scale of genocidal acts, and questions whether the United Nations can ever play an effective and impartial role.[50]

If there are difficulties in prosecuting genocidal killings, then there will be even more reticence and enumerated obstacles to prosecuting genocidal rape – because of traditional and prevailing dismissals of sexual crimes as indicated in the two quotes at the opening of this chapter.

Yet there have been moves indicating some (albeit limited) preparedness to indict, prosecute and punish perpetrators of rape in genocides. Human Rights Watch provided a summary report regarding the international tribunals and crimes of sexual violence, noting that acts of sexual violence fall within the jurisdiction of the International Criminal Tribunals for both Yugoslavia (including Kosovo) (ICTY) and Rwanda (ICTR). By March 1999, the ICTY had indicted 27 individuals in relation to 130 individual crimes that involved either rape or sexual assault. The jurisprudence of the international criminal tribunals does include rape prosecuted as genocide.[51]

The case of Jean-Paul Akayesu, who was found guilty of genocide – including genocidal rape – by the ICTR in September 2 1998, was a breakthrough in the prosecution of rape in genocide. Human Rights Watch issued a statement saying: "The verdict is the first handed down by the Rwandan Tribunal; the first conviction for genocide by an international court; the first time an international court has punished sexual violence in a civil war; and the first time that rape was found to be an act of genocide to destroy a group." HRW spokesperson Regan Ralph, an authority on violence against women, continued, "Rape is a serious crime like any other. That's always been true on paper, but now international courts are finally acting on it."[52]

In February 2001, in another historic court ruling, Bosnian Serbs were convicted by the ICTY for rape, torture and enslavement. This provoked Regan Ralph to comment: "This decision is historic because it puts those who rape and sexually enslave women on notice that they will not get away with these heinous crimes."[53]

However, the cases against the Bosnian Serbs did not make a direct link between rape and genocide in the way it had been done in the Akayesu case.

Even now with the indictment of Slobodan Milosevic there is still no further, solid recognition that rape of itself can be a genocidal act.This latter case, does, however, show that heads of sovereign states can be brought to account – even if one may acknowledge that world politics leading to this happening are complex and probably involve a variety of motivations.

In all, the difficulties in prosecuting those guilty of genocide are acknowledged. But, difficulty in implementing prosecution should not be equated with any logical or ethical reason to avoid acknowledging, naming, and increasing awareness of genocide. This is true of genocide by direct slaying or genocide by rape, which has the same outcome.

Closing

So, why does it matter whether rape can be genocidal? It matters because it needs to be recognised that it is possible for genocide to be committed by means other than campaigns of mass slaying. Genocide by rape is and has been a potent form of genocide – whether or not it involves accompanying or parallel campaigns of slaying. Recognising that genocide by rape is a reality matters if the Convention matters because Article IV says, "Persons committing genocide or any of the other acts enumerated in Article III shall be punished, whether they are constitutional rulers, public officials or private individuals." It matters because, given the lack of interest in prosecuting crimes of sexual violence against women more generally, it is also possible that genocide by rape could go unnoticed, not condemned, not prosecuted or unpunished, and that few resources would be allocated to proactive strategies of prevention.

References

1 A Serbian Orthodox priest, interview with author, Zagreb, December 1992

2 Julia Hall, lawyer with Human Rights Watch, in an interview reported by Alexandra Poolos, 'Human Rights Advocates Say Rape is War Crime', Radio Free Europe, 25 May 1999

3 *Geneva Convention, Protocol II*, Article 4 (20) (e), 1949

4 Brenda Fitzpatrick, *Rape of Women in War*, World Council of Churches, Geneva, 1992

5 United Nations Economic and Social Council, 'Rape and Abuse of Women in the Territory of the Former Yugoslavia', *Commission on Human Rights Resolution 1993/8*, 23 February 2001

6 United Nations General Assembly, 'Rape and Abuse of Women in the Areas of Armed Conflict in the Former Yugoslavia', General Assembly *Resolution 1994/205*, 6 March 1995

7 Text of the 1948 Genocide Convention quoted in George J. Andreopoulos, *Genocide: Conceptual and Historical Dimensions*, University of Pennsylvania Press, Philadelphia, 1997

8 Frank Chalk, 'Redefining Genocide', and Israel W. Charny, 'Toward a Generic Definition of Genocide', in Andreopoulos, *ibid.*

9 Peter J. Stoett, 'This Age of Genocide: Conceptual and Institutional Implications', Deakin Reader in the *International Journal*, Vol. 1, No. 3, Summer 1995

10 *Geneva Convention*, Article II (b)

11 International Criminal Tribunal for Rwanda, *Summary of the Judgement in Jean-Paul Akayesu Case*, ICTR-96-4-T, paragraph 51, 2 September 1998, http://www.un.org/ictr/english/singledocs/ipa_summary.html

12 M. Cherif Bassiouni, *Rape and Sexual Assault: Final Report of the United Nations Commission of Experts Established Pursuant to Security Council Resolution 780 (1992)*, Annex IX, United Nations Security Council, 28 December 1994

[13] European Council Investigative Mission into the Treatment of Muslim Women in the Former Yugoslavia, *Report to the European Council Foreign Ministers*, 28 January 1993, paragraph 14

[14] Norma Von Ragenfeld-Feldman, 'The Victimization of Women: Rape and the Reporting of Rape in Bosnia-Herzegovina, 1992–1993', presented at Fifth Annual Interdisciplinary German Studies Conference, 15–16 March 1997

[15] Bassiouni, *op. cit.*

[16] Human Rights Watch, *Bosnia and Hercegovina, 'A Closed Dark Place': Past and Present Human Rights Abuses in Foca* Vol. 10, No. 6 (D), 1998

[17] Peter Maas, *Love Thy Neighbour: A Story of War*, Papermac, Macmillan, London, 1996, pp. 51–52, 12–13, 5–7, 53–54

[18] Alison Des Forges, *Leave None to Tell the Story*, Human Rights Watch, New York, March 1999, p. 1

[19] Binaifer Nowrojee, *Shattered Lives: Sexual Violence during the Rwandan Genocide and its Aftermath*, Human Rights Watch, New York, 1996

[20] Comment from a woman staff member of Médecins sans Frontieres to the author, in Ngara in 1994. It was a comment echoed many times by a variety of Tanzanian and European personnel dealing with the refugees.

[21] International Criminal Tribunal for Rwanda, *op. cit.*, paragraph 19

[22] Helen Fein, 'Genocide, Terror, Life Integrity, and War Crimes', in Andreopoulos, *op. cit.*, pp. 96, 102

[23] Martina E. Vandenburg, 'The Aftermath: Ongoing Issues Facing Kosovar Albanian Women', in *Federal Republic of Yugoslavia: Kosovo – Rape as a Weapon of 'Ethnic Cleansing'*, Vol. 12, No. 3, Human Rights Watch, Women's Rights Division, March 2000

[24] Nowrojee, *op. cit.*, p. 2

[25] *ibid.*

[26] *ibid.*, p. 3

[27] *ibid.*, p. 3

[28] Fitzpatrick, *op. cit.*, p. 20

[29] Bassiouni, 'Annex IV, The policy of Ethnic Cleansing,' in *Final Report*, *op. cit.*

[30] Nowrojee, *op. cit.*, 'Introduction'

[31] Judgement of Jean-Paul Akaseyu, *op. cit.* paragraph 27

[32] Stoett, *op. cit.*, p 602

[33] Andreopoulos, *op. cit.*, text of the 1948 Genocide Convention, Article II

[34] Judgement of Jean-Paul Akaseyu, *op. cit.*, paragraphs 37 and 38

[35] Bassiouni, Annexe IX, *op. cit.*, p 9

[36] Fein, *op. cit.*, p 97

[37] Bassiouni, *op. cit.*, pp 8, 9

[38] Human Rights Watch, 'Bosnia and Hercegovina. 'A Closed Dark Place' Past and Present Human Rights Abuses in Foca', *op. cit.*

[39] United Nations ECOSOC Resolution 1993/8, *op. cit.*

[40] United Nations General Assembly Resolution 1994/205, *op. cit.*

[41] Fitzpatrick, *op. cit.*, pp. 21, 20

[42] Brenda Fitzpatrick, *Kosovo: the Women and Children*, World Vision Australia, Burwood East, 1999, pp. 14–15

[43] Nowrojee, *op. cit.*, pp. 19, 20, 25

[44] Bassiouni, *op. cit.*, pp. 7–8

[45] Nowrojee, *op. cit.*, p. 11

[46] Gerard Prunier, 'Genocide and Renewed War (6 April – 14 June 1994)', Deakin Reading 27 in Gerard Prunier, *The Rwanda Crisis: History of a Genocide*, Columbia University Press, New York, 1995, pp. 239, 244

[47] Des Forges, *op. cit.*, p. 564

[48] Fein, *op. cit.*, p. 105

[49] Andreopolous, *op. cit.*, pp. 3, 18

[50] Stoett, *op. cit.*, pp. 612–614

[51] Human Rights Watch, 'Kosovo Backgrounder: Sexual Violence as International Crime,' 10 May 1999

[52] Human Rights Watch, 'Human Rights Watch Applauds Rwanda Rape Verdict,' 2 September 1998

[53] Human Rights Watch, 'Bosnia: Landmark Verdicts for Rape, Torture and Sexual Enslavement,' 22 February 2001

Violence against women in Europe

Sylvia Mpaayei

Introduction: The cost of silence

Violence against women is a hidden evil in almost all societies – a secret, silent problem in many homes and cities around the world. Many women suffer silently, too afraid to share what they experience because they feel ashamed about what has happened to them. Compounding the problem is that women do not want to humiliate those close to them by divulging that they were abused.

The tragedy is the cost of this nearly invisible societal "disease" – the cost of ill health. Studies exploring violence and health consistently report negative and far-reaching effects. The true extent is difficult to determine because of the largely invisible nature of the crimes. Physical health outcomes of violence against women include injury, unwanted pregnancy, gynaecological problems, permanent disabilities, asthma and self-injurious behaviours. The mental health outcomes are even more daunting and include depression, fear, anxiety, low self-esteem, sexual dysfunction, eating disorders, obsessive-compulsive disorder and post-traumatic stress disorder. The fatal outcomes are often suicide, murder, maternal mortality and HIV/AIDS.[1]

Violence is described as "intentional use of physical force or power (threatened or actual) against a person, resulting in injury, death or psychological harm." It is estimated that 20–50% of women in the world have experienced physical or sexual abuse sometime in their lives.[2]

Violence against women occurs in many forms and in all places – at home, in the workplace and in the community. Numerous studies clearly show that the most pervasive form of gender-based abuse is carried out in homes against women by their intimate male partners. Rape and other forms of sexually coercive relationships are also widely prevalent.[3]

Psychological and emotional abuse, such as constant belittling, intimidation and humiliating treatment, also put women at risk of depression, suicide attempt, chronic pain syndrome and psychosomatic disorders.[4]

If violence has such a negative impact on women's health, why are women silent? Women are often silent because they do not know what alternatives are available to them. Many do not have systems of justice and governance to support them and to set them free from the violence they face, but even where such systems are in place, some women remain silent. Women dependent on spouses for an income are afraid to leave the only form of security they know. Women are often cowed into silence due to fear: the fear of repeated or increased violence against them by the people that abuse them. Women are silent from shame, the humiliation of sharing what violence has done to their minds and bodies.

In Europe, as elsewhere, violence against women is an obstacle to the achievement of gender equality, development and peace, and of course to the human rights of women.

Violence in relationships

Europe today is faced with a rising number of cases of violence against women:[5]

- At least one in five women in the European Union (EU) experienced abuse by their intimate male partner, with some 95% of all acts of violence taking place in the home.[6]
- In the Netherlands, data for 1989 revealed that 21% of women questioned in a survey had been subjected to physical violence by a male partner or ex-partner, at some time during their lives. Some 13% of women were experiencing sexual/and or physical violence at the time of the survey.

- Information from Belgium in 1998 showed that "Partners are the most dangerous perpetrators; they are over-represented in relation to moderately severe and serious acts of violence." In about 48% of cases of violence against women, the perpetrator was a male partner.
- In Finland, 40% of adult women were victims of physical or sexual violence inflicted by men, or were threatened with violence, after their 15th birthday. Moreover, data for 1998 revealed that 22% of married or cohabiting women experienced violence or threats thereof at the hands of their current male partner, 9% of them during the previous year.
- A national survey conducted in France in 2000 indicated that 10% of women were subjected to violence from their partner during the last year; 18% had experienced physical violence and about 11% sexual violence since the age of 18; and 9% of women had experienced rape or an attempted rape, almost 3% before the age of 18. Also in France, of the 25,000 cases of rape actually taking place every year, only 8,000 are officially reported to the police.[7]
- Statistics collected by ROKS, the main women's organisation in Sweden, showed an increase in the number of rape cases reported: 885 cases in 1980 compared to 1,998 in 1998.[8]

Europe overall continues to struggle to adhere to international standards on issues of violence against women. This is illustrated in the concerns documented in the Reporting Committee of the Convention on the Elimination of All Forms of Discrimination Against Women (CEDAW).

Violence and trafficking in Eastern Europe

Among the major recent concerns of the CEDAW Reporting Committee have been the failure of the Government of Armenia to address violence against women; and the expansion of trafficking in women in Romania as a country of both origin and transit. There is also an absence of legislation criminalising domestic violence, including marital rape, in Romania.[9]

The situation for Albanian women is no different. Domestic violence has worsened in recent years and remains behind closed doors, supported by tradition. The Albanian civil code has no provisions to ensure that a person who is believed to be in danger has the right to demand a temporary court decision to prevent the violence. Only 5% of cases of domestic violence are brought to court.[10]

In addition, the trafficking of women and girls in Albania continues to be a major problem. Save the Children carried out a detailed study on trafficking of under-18 year olds (and also women) from Albania, concluding that thousands of women and children have been lied to or abducted outright, and forced into the commercial sex trade abroad. The study found that this recruitment still occurs on a daily basis. According to the report, at least 60% of Albanians trafficked for prostitution are children; the number in some areas is as high as 80%. Of those trafficked, most (60%) are deceived into the sex trade, and 35% are abducted. Furthermore, in some rural areas, up to 90% of girls over the age of 14 have stopped attending school due to fear of being trafficked.[11]

The International Organization for Migration (IOM) and International Catholic Migration Commission (ICMC) report on trafficking in women in Albania sheds new light on the levels of violence and of sexual exploitation suffered by victims. The report is based on the testimonies of 125 women who were assisted last year by IOM and ICMC. It shows that 73% of the victims, mostly Moldovans and Romanians, were cheated by traffickers into believing they were going to Europe to get jobs as waitresses, nannies or au pairs. The report says that 18% of victims had been kidnapped and 32% had been raped and beaten into submission. A further 73% said they suffered intimidation and confinement. The evidence in the reports demonstrates that trafficking in and through Albania of women and children remains a major problem.[12]

Domestic violence: a major challenge

The greatest violence problem in Europe is clearly violence in the home. In June 1999 a survey[13] was conducted by the European Commission to examine what Europeans thought about issues relating to domestic violence against women. A total of 16,179 people were polled in over 15 countries (an average of around 1,000 per country).

European attitudes

The Eurobarometer survey showed that 89% of Europeans had heard of domestic violence (including through the media). Some 62% of Europeans considered domestic violence against women to be "unacceptable in all circumstances and always punishable by law," while 32% who considered it "unacceptable in all circumstances but not always punishable by law." Only 2% said it was "acceptable in certain circumstances" and 0.7% that it was "acceptable in all circumstances." One European in two (50%) thought that domestic violence was fairly common. Sexual violence against women was rated as very serious by 90% of Europeans, physical violence by 87%, psychological violence by 65%, restricted freedom by 64% and threats of violence by 58%.

When asked whether they knew of any women who had been victims of some form of domestic violence, a scant 11% responded that they knew of someone where they worked or studied, only 18% in their neighbourhood or immediate area, and barely 19% in their circle of friends and family. This would indicate that the culture of silence persists. Women are facing violence but they remain silent. A silence that must be broken.

Perceived causes

Concerning causes of domestic violence of women, survey respondents cited a range of factors:

- An overwhelming majority viewed alcohol (96%) or drugs (94%) as causes
- 79% identified unemployment, and 75% poverty or social exclusion, as causes
- 73% cited "having oneself been a victim of some form of domestic violence"
- 64% believed there was such a thing as a genetic predisposition to violence
- 64% cited the way women are viewed by men, and 59% the way power is shared between the sexes
- 57% cited a low level of education

and

- less than 50% of respondents identified harmful effects of the media, religious beliefs, or the provocative behaviour of women as causes of domestic violence.[14]

Favoured solutions

For solutions to the problem of violence against women, 95% of people thought that punishing perpetrators served a useful purpose and 91% thought tougher enforcement of existing laws did. About 91% thought teaching young people about mutual respect, while 89% recommended providing a freephone number for women seeking help and advice. Other responses included: information leaflets written for perpetrators (86%), tougher laws (86%), laws to prevent sexual discrimination (85%), and campaigns to raise public awareness (84%). Additionally, 81% of respondents thought a small card with emergency contact numbers would help; 78% felt that teaching police officers about women's rights is needed, and 65% were in favour of rehabilitating domestic violence perpetrators.

Rehabilitation for perpetrators

While only 39% thought there were special laws in their country concerning rehabilitation of perpetrators, 42% thought there was no legislation on prevention of domestic violence against women. However, 45% thought there were laws on "social support for victims of domestic violence 51% on "legal support for victims" and 58% on punishment of perpetrators. Some 79% were unaware of any policies or measures put forward by the European Union to combat domestic violence against women.

Assistance for victims

At least 96% of Europeans felt that family and friends should help women affected by domestic violence. Some 93% felt that social services, 91% medical services, 90% the police, 86% the state, 83% solicitors and barristers, 80% charitable or voluntary organisations, 65% religious organisations and 64% the media do, or should, help abused women.

Domestic violence in the UK

Domestic violence currently wrecks the lives of thousands of women and children in the United Kingdom (UK). It is a major cause of family distress and social exclusion, and it is rarely a one-off event. One violent incident tends to lead to another, and such incidents often increase in frequency and severity over time, sometimes only ending when someone is killed. Typically, the violence begins from a pattern of abusive and controlling behaviour, which can take a number of forms. Some are directly or indirectly physical, such as assault, rape, destruction of property and threats. Some are non-physical, such as destructive criticism, pressure tactics, belittling, breaking trust, isolation, oppressive control of finances and harassment.

Alarming statistics

People experience domestic violence regardless of their social group, class, age, race, disability, sexuality and lifestyle. Research studies have found that one in four women in the UK experiences domestic violence at some time in her life.[15] Some of the alarming statistics on domestic violence in the UK:

- In any one day, nearly 7,000 women and children are sheltering from violence in refuges.[16]
- 70% of children staying with mothers in refuges have been abused by their father.[17]
- Every minute in the UK, the police receive a call from the public for assistance for domestic violence (an estimated 1,300 calls each day or over 570,000 each year).[18]
- The estimated total costs of providing advice, support and assistance for those facing domestic violence in Greater London are £278 million (US $395 million) per year.[19]
- The total number of incidents of domestic violence in 1995 was estimated at 6.6 million.[20]
- In 1999, 37% of women murder victims were killed by present or former partners, compared to 6% of men. This totals approximately 92 women a year – one every three days or two women per week.[21]
- Women who are physically abused report an average of four injuries a year.[22]
- Domestic violence is a factor in at least one-quarter of suicide attempts by women.[23]
- About 20% of young men and 10% of young women think violence against women is acceptable.[24]
- The psychological impact of domestic violence has been found to have parallels with the impact of torture and imprisonment of hostages.[25]
- Domestic violence often starts or intensifies during pregnancy and is associated with increased rates of miscarriage, low birth weight, premature birth, and foetal injury or death.[26]
- A 1996 British Crime Survey revealed that 12% of women with disabilities aged 16–29 had experienced domestic violence in 1995. This compares with 8.2% of non-disabled women of the same age.[27]
- Safe accommodation is a primary concern for those fleeing domestic violence. There are about 418 refuges (shelters) for victims of domestic violence in England and 45 in Wales.[28]
- Of all types of crimes reported to the British Crime Survey in 2000, more than one in 20 were classified as domestic violence; this accounts for almost a quarter (23%) of all violent crime. It is also the least likely crime to be reported to the police (only one-third of incidences were reported in 2000). No other type of crime has a rate of repeat victimisation as high.[29]

The British Government is responding to the alarm-

ing data on domestic abuse with various initiatives. In 1994, an official Interdepartmental Working Party on Domestic Violence was set up to promote a co-ordinated response to the problem at national and local levels. In particular a working party considered ways of improving services of victims, encouraging local co-ordination and raising awareness of domestic violence.[30]

A ministerial group was also established to take forward work in this area. In 1997, the Government appointed for the first time two Ministers for Women, supported by a Women's Unit. This unit has been instrumental in the development of a programme of measures to promote women's issues and rights, in collaboration with the Home Office and other departments. The document *Living Without Fear: An integrated approach to tackling violence against women*, published in June 1999, sets out government strategy framework in relation to violence against women and offers examples of good practice from around the country.[31]

In January 1999, the Government launched a new domestic violence publicity/awareness campaign for England and Wales under the title "Break the Chain." A leaflet titled *Break the Chain: What you can do about domestic violence* was distributed to the general public by the police, courts and others; it emphasises that domestic violence is not acceptable, sets out the sources of help available to survivors, and advises survivors' friends on how they can help.[32]

A report on policing domestic violence using effective organisational structures was commissioned by the Home Office and published in January 1999. It found that 38 police forces had published a domestic violence policy document, but that 65% of operational Domestic Violence Officers (DVOs), 48% of line managers for DVOs and 39% of policy makers within the police felt there was a significant gap between policy and practice.[33]

The UK Home Affairs Select Committee produced a report in 1993 that defined domestic violence as: "any form of physical, sexual or emotional abuse which takes place within the context of a close relationship. In most cases, the relationship will be between partners or ex-partners."[34] From April 1999, a new definition of domestic violence came into effect for use in police returns to the HMIC (Her Majesty's Inspectorate of Constabulary); this definition is intended for statistical purposes only and is designed to allow easier comparison of domestic violence statistics between police forces; it also gives a better understanding of the nature of information being collected:

> "The term 'domestic violence' shall be understood to mean any violence between current or former partners in an intimate relationship, wherever and whenever it occurs. The violence may include physical, sexual, emotional or financial abuse."[35]

Addressing offending behaviour is also a priority. An evaluation was done of two court-ordered treatment programmes for men found guilty of violence against female partners ("CHANGE" and "Lothian Domestic Violence Probation Programme"). The evaluation compared treatment programmes with more traditional criminal justice sanctions. Though based on a relatively small sample, the research found that all criminal justice interventions (fine, probation, prison) appeared to have positive effects on the behaviour of men convicted of violence against their female partner.[36]

Facing the challenge across Europe

In recent years, some progress has been made in Europe to address violence against women. Since 1996 many initiatives have been taken, both at European Community level, by individual Member States, and by non-governmental bodies including the Church.

A main objective of the European Commission is to ensure that the issue of violence against women, including the fight against trafficking in women, is put high on the political agenda of the European Union.[37] The objectives of the European Community's activities are:

- to prevent and eliminate violence against women

- to study the causes and consequences of violence against women, and the effectiveness of preventive measures

and

- to eliminate trafficking in women and assist victims of forced prostitution and trafficking.[38]

Violence in the form of trafficking in women was specifically addressed in 1996 with a *Communication* on trafficking in women[39] that stated the main objectives as increasing cooperation and coordination among the Member States and EU accession applicant countries, and providing greater protection for victims of trafficking, especially those who are prepared to testify as witnesses.[40]

In the *Second Communication on further Actions in the Fight against Trafficking in Women* in December 1998, the Commission sought to better understand current conditions, identify gaps and recommend a number of new objectives, which included:[41]

- to ensure that the question of trafficking remains high on the political agenda
- to reinforce international and European cooperation including both governments and NGOs in countries of origin, transit and destination
- to strengthen a multi-disciplinary approach focusing on prevention, research, law-enforcement and effective sentencing of traffickers, as well as on support to victims
- to address a clear message to candidate countries, in the context of the accession process, on the necessity of national measures and cooperation with the EU on the issue.

Through the Joint Action of February 1997,[42] the Member States agreed to review their national legislation with a view to criminalising a number of offences, and to introduce specific and serious sanctions with regard to trafficking in human beings for the purpose of sexual exploitation.[43]

A Community Programme called "STOP" was set up in 1996 to reinforce cooperation against trafficking in women and children. As a result of this, a number of trans-national projects addressing the issue of trafficking in women have received support. This was followed by the DAPHNE initiative (1979–1999) to support and promote close cooperation with and among NGOs active in this field, to improve statistics and information on violence against women and children, and to encourage preventive measures to strengthen the protection of victims of violence. The new DAPHNE programme (2000–2003; COM (98) 726) with a budget of 20 million euros (or US $19.6 million), permits multi-annual actions, is open to public bodies in addition to NGOs, and will be opened to the applicant states and the EEA/AFTA countries.[44]

Europe's "Violence Against Women" campaign

In January 1999 the European Commission launched the European campaign on Violence Against Women with a budget of approximately 4 million euros (about US $3.5). The main objectives of this campaign were to promote public awareness and to find ways to prevent domestic violence. The campaign was an occasion for numerous initiatives at national and local level in every Member State, such as the promotion of nation-wide campaigns and action plans to combat violence against women. One major result is a greater recognition of violence against women as a serious and permanent problem.[45]

"Combating violence against disabled people" was the theme chosen for the campaign's 1999 international conference on the European Day of Disabled People, 3 December. The theme's specific pertinence to women with disabilities was underlined.[46]

At the campaign's official close, at its international conference in Lisbon in May 2000, the Presidency called on the Council, the Commission and the Member States to make a solemn commitment (see endnote 37 for a clarification of terms):

- to combat all forms of violence against women through the adoption of legal, administrative and other provisions
- to ensure a study on violence and its prevention

- to ensure the protection, assistance and compensation of the victims
- to coordinate a Violence against Women Year around 2001–2003
- to set up a unit (within the Commission) to maintain the momentum of work on the issue

and

- to present a communication on violence against women. [47]

Strengthening women to promote peace

The European Community also supports conflict prevention schemes, is active in confidence-building measures to restore peace and promotes the observance of international humanitarian law by all parties to a conflict. Recognising the important role of women in the peace process, it has supported schemes covering and promoting women's interests in the peace process in the Balkan and Mediterranean regions and projects promoting women's political and electoral participation. It has also provided psychological help and counselling for women war victims in and from Bosnia. NGOs that have acquired experience in dealing with violence against women in conflict situations have been supported to pass on their experience to other NGOs through training seminars. The European Community also supports projects to help women who have suffered female-specific human rights abuses. [48]

The church

The church has also made some progress in addressing the issue of violence against women. To take just one example, the Methodist Church in the UK has a Women's Network which has a Women and Violence Task Group. This project was established to work from 2000 to 2002 to raise awareness on violence in three specific contexts: domestic violence, the trafficking of women, and female genital mutilation; and to challenge the Methodist Church itself to address the issue of violence against women and work to achieve change.

Among its numerous accomplishments in the last two years, this group initiated and supported the "Way Forward Project," a programme of research into domestic violence by Dr. Lorraine Radford and Cecilia Cappel of Roehampton Surrey University and funded by the Southlands Methodist Centre. The research acknowledged that although women are most often the victims, domestic violence is an important issue that all members of the church, men and women, need to accept and confront.

The British Methodist Conference (the denomination's major decision- and policy-making body in the UK), at its annual Conference in June 2002, approved the recommendations of the "Way Forward Project." The recommendations included appointing a task group to include members of the Methodist Women's Network, the church's Family and Personal Relationships Committee and its Faith and Order Committee, to manage, direct and monitor further work and study in four areas:

- *Theology:* developing theological understandings of marriage, the family, violence and forgiveness
- *Policy:* developing policy for responding to domestic violence
- *Practice:* developing practice guidelines

and

- *Training:* in cooperation with, and recognising the expertise of, other agencies working in this field, to identify and develop appropriate training on domestic violence

all of which are to be used throughout the Methodist Church.

It is encouraging to see examples of the Christian church making progress towards addressing the fundamental issues that women battle with when confronted with situations of violence. [49]

Practical support for women

Awareness-raising among women themselves remains a challenge. Women's reactions to violence depend on their level of awareness and education;

capability to fight to protect themselves; support received from parents, children and others; economic situation; and information they have on existing civil services.[50]

Some of the measures taken across the world to help women help themselves have been:[51]

- support groups, where women can share their experiences and be helped to cope with their violent experiences
- local community involvement in the reporting and rebuking of violent husbands
- women's police stations providing a more committed and concerned response to crimes against women
- courses in non-violent parenting and conflict resolution for adults and children
- legal literacy programmes and free legal advice encouraging battered women to press charges

and

- sensitivity training for health professionals and the police, and their adoption of new protocols for dealing with the victims of domestic violence.

Closing

Progress is slowly being made to address issues of violence facing women in Europe. Women facing violence will not always report the crimes committed against them. The culture of silence persists in many societies, and within the hearts and minds of many women. Our challenge is to support women facing violence by empowering them to make wise decisions about their own health, to report the crimes of violence against them and combat the culture of silence, and to nurture hope of a better future for themselves.

References

1 'Women's Health, Development and Family Reproductive Health'. *Violence against Women*, WHO Consultation, World Health Organisation, Geneva, 5–7 February 1996, pp. 10–11

2 UNICEF, 'Domestic Violence against Women and Girls', *Innocenti Digest*, No. 6, June 2000, p. 4

3 NGO Forum for Health, *Violence and Health: Proceedings of a Symposium*, World Health Organisation, Geneva, 14 May 2001, p. 25

4 UNICEF, *op. cit.*, pp. 7, 10, 11

5 All bullet points are quoted from European Women's Lobby, *EU Gender Equality Policies. Persistence of Gender Inequalities – Facts and Figures in 1995 to 2000*, February 2001, http://www.womenlobby.org/

6 European Women's Lobby, 'Unveiling the Hidden Data on Domestic Violence in the EU, 1999,' quoted in *ibid.*

7 European Women's Lobby, *op. cit.*

8 National Organisation for Women's and Young Women's Shelters in Sweden (Riksorganisationen för kvinnojourer och tjejjourer i Sverige), *How it all began*, http://www.roks.se/english/beginning.html

9 CEDAW, 'Most Recent Concerns of the Reporting Committees on the Convention on the Elimination of All Forms of Discrimination against Women'; see http://www.un.org/womenwatch/daw/cedaw/29sess.htm for details of forthcoming CEDAW session.

10 UNICEF, *Mapping out Existing Information on Domestic Violence in Albania*, October 2000, p. 2

11 Save the Children, 'Save the Children Albania', press release, 17 April 2001, cited in the research report *Third Country National Trafficking Victims in Albania*, International Organization of Migration and International Catholic Migration Commission, 2001

12 Save the Children, *ibid.*

13 Eurobarometer 51.0, *Europeans and their Views on*

Domestic Violence against Women, and European Commission Directorate-General, *Information, Communication, Culture and Audiovisual Media*, June 1999, p. 1

[14] *ibid.*

[15] *Domestic Violence: Break the Chain. Multi-Agency Guidance for Addressing Domestic Violence*, Home Office, London, 2000

[16] Women's Aid Federation of England, *Domestic Violence Statistical Factsheet No. 1*, Bristol, UK, August 2001

[17] L. Bowker, M. Arbitell & J. McFerron, cited in Women's Aid Federation of England, *Domestic Violence Statistical Factsheet No. 3*, August 1999. (Note: date and number of "Factsheets" don't necessarily correspond.)

[18] Professor E. Stanko, 'The Day to Count: A Snapshot of the Impact of Domestic Violence in the UK', *Criminal Justice*, 1:2, 2000; cited in Women's Aid Federation of England, 2001, *op. cit.*

[19] Stanko, 'Counting the Costs. London: Crime Concern'; cited in Women's Aid Federation of England, *ibid.*

[20] *Government Policy Around Domestic Violence*, Home Office, London, 1999

[21] *Criminal Statistics England and Wales 1999*, Home Office, London, 2000; cited in Women's Aid Federation of England, 2001, *op. cit.*

[22] J. Mooney, *The Hidden Figure: Domestic Violence in North London*, Middlesex University Centre of Criminology, London, 1993; cited in Women's Aid Federation of England, *Domestic Violence Statistical Factsheet No. 2*, August 2001

[23] E. Stark & A. Flitcraft. *Women at Risk: Domestic Violence and Women's Health* (London: Sage), 1996, cited in Women's Aid Federation of England, Factsheet No. 2, *ibid.*

[24] Zero Tolerance Charitable Trust, cited in Women's Aid Federation of England, Factsheet No. 1, *op. cit.*

[25] P. Graham, *et al.*, 'Survivors of Terror: Battered Women, Hostages and the Stockholm Syndrome', in K. Yllo & M. Bograd (eds), *Feminist Perspectives on Wife Abuse*, London: Sage, 1988, cited in Women's Aid Federation of England, Factsheet No. 2, *op. cit.*

[26] G. C. Mezey, 'Domestic Violence in Pregnancy', in S. Bewley, *et al., Violence Against Women*, London: RCOG, 1997; cited in Women's Aid Federation of England, Factsheet No. 2

[27] C. Mirrlees-Black, *Domestic Violence: BCS Self-Completion Questionnaire*, London: Home Office, 1999: cited in Women's Aid Federation of England, Factsheet No. 1, *op. cit*

[28] *Government Policy Around Domestic Violence*, 1999, *loc. cit.*

[29] *The British Crime Survey: England and Wales*, Home Office, London, 2000; cited in Women's Aid Federation of England, Factsheet No. 1, *op. cit.*

[30] *Government Policy Around Domestic Violence*, *op. cit.*

[31] *ibid.*

[32] *ibid.*

[33] *ibid.*

[34] *ibid.*

[35] *ibid.*

[36] *ibid.*

[37] *European Union Annual Report on Human Rights, 2000*, p. 23, http://europa.eu.int/comm/external_relations/human_rights/doc/report_00_en.pdf

For the interest of readers:

- The *European Community (EC)* was established in 1956 by the Treaty in Rome. Its central feature is the Single Market, but other activities have been added including development cooperation. It is served by a number of institutions, including the European Commission, the Council of Ministers and the European Parliament.
- The *European Union (EU)* was established in 1992

by the Maastricht Treaty. It comprises what are known as three pillars: the EC (as above); inter-governmental cooperation (i.e., between national governments) in foreign and security policy; and inter-governmental cooperation in justice and home affairs. Although the same institutions serve the three pillars, the roles of the Commission and Parliament in the two inter-governmental pillars are much smaller. Policies and actions for development cooperation come mainly under the first pillar, though competence is shared in certain areas (e.g. conflict) between the first two pillars.

- The *Council of the European Union*, formerly known as the Council of Ministers, is the main legislative and decision-making institution in the EU. The Council is composed of ministers who represent the national governments of the 15 Member States. It provides a forum for the Member States to legislate for the Union, set its political objectives and coordinate national policies. Council members are politically accountable to their national parliaments, and the Council is where they assert their interests and reach compromises.
- The *European Council* decides the major policy guidelines. It meets at the level of heads of State/Government. Also known as summits, these are regular meetings whose role is to provide overall political direction to the EU and to resolve the problems that have proved intractable at the Council level. These summits mainly involve high-profile decision-making and changes in direction of EU policy. They are held at least twice a year either in Brussels or in the country holding the presidency. The President of the Commission attends, as do foreign ministers.
- The *European Commission* does much of the day-to-day work in the European Union and is the driving force in the Union's institutional system. It is an independent body appointed by the Member States to act as a neutral guardian of their shared interests. It ensures that the provisions of the Treaties and the decisions of the institutions are properly implemented. The Commission drafts policies and legislation and represents the Community interest. It does not, however, take any decisions on EU policies and priorities, as this is the prerogative of the Council and in some cases, the European Parliament.

[38] European Commission, *Implementation by the European Community of the Platform for Action Adopted at the Fourth World Conference on Women in Beijing 1995*, Working Document from the Commission Services, May 2000, p. 18

[39] European Commission, *Communication on Trafficking in Women*, COM (96) 567, 1996

[40] European Commission, *op. cit.*, p. 18

[41] *ibid.*, p. 19

[42] European Union, *Joint Action* (OJ L 63 of 4 1997, pp. 2–6)

[43] European Commission, *op. cit.*, p. 18

[44] *ibid.*, pp. 18–19.

[45] *European Union Annual Report on Human Rights, 2000*, *op. cit.*, p. 23

[46] European Commission, *op. cit.*, p. 20

[47] European Union, *op. cit.*

[48] European Commission, *op. cit.*, p. 21

[49] Women's Network, Methodist Church in the UK, http://www.methodist.org.uk/womensnetwork/wv_project.htm; or contact: womens.network@methodistchurch.org.uk

[50] UNICEF, *Mapping out Existing Information on Domestic Violence in Albania*, *loc. cit.*, p. 2

[51] All bullet points quoted from World Health Organisation, *Violence against Women in Families*, information pack, July 1997, http://www.who.int/violence_injury_prevention/vaw/infopack.htm

Family and sexual violence in Papua New Guinea

Frieda Kana

Introduction

Violence against women and children is a growing problem in Papua New Guinea that needs to be urgently addressed. This concern was expressed by Papua New Guinea's Family and Sexual Violence Action Committee during a workshop in Port Moresby in September 2001.

In Papua New Guinea (PNG) the problem is known as "family and sexual violence," but the majority of victims are female and the majority of perpetrators male. Violence against women is, after all, violence against families. It also affects the economic contribution of PNG women to the development of the nation. It is both a development issue and a crucial human rights issue.

Family and sexual violence is a phenomenon that has its roots in various areas; in some cases it is linked with family poverty. But it is a fact of life in PNG that needs immediate attention.

The PNG Government has made a number of international and national commitments to eliminate this human rights abuse. Unfortunately, no policy framework or plan of action has yet been put in place.

The Family Violence Action Committee, under the umbrella of the Institute of National Affairs, has been organising and mobilising non-governmental organisations (NGOs) and churches to urge the Government to seriously consider legislating against family and sexual violence. The introduction of a legislative bill in Parliament on 11 October 2001 was an important step towards this, but only a bill relating to incest (introduced by Lady Carol Kidu, Member for Port Moresby South and now Minister for Welfare and Social Development) was passed by the Parliament, in 2002.

A primary source of data on violence against women in PNG used in this chapter is *Family and Sexual Violence in PNG: An Integrated Long-Term Strategy* (LTS). The LTS was developed during a six-week study conducted in March and April 2001 by the Family Violence Action Committee of the Consultative Implementation and Monitoring Committee and funded by the British High Commission. A two-person team gathered information from written materials and consultations with stakeholders in Port Moresby, East New Britain, Morobe, Simbu Eastern Highlands and East Sepik provinces.

The report from the Family Violence Action Committee states that there are no national statistics for cases of family and sexual violence compiled from the records of agencies providing medical, legal and social services to victims. Police crime reports do provide national statistics, but do not cover domestic violence, sexual harassment or child abuse. Other agency statistics also give only a very partial picture, because reported cases represent a tiny proportion of what really occurs in the community.

Domestic violence

The most extensive form of family and sexual violence in PNG is domestic violence. This usually refers to violence between husbands and wives, though it can also include violence between other members of a domestic group. In reality, most domestic violence is wife beating – a phenomenon so common in PNG that it has been used in courts as proof of marriage. (In one court case, a government minister's defence against charges of raping a young girl in his household was that he considered her to be one of his wives.)

Domestic violence was extensively researched by the Law Reform Commission (LRC) in preparation for its parliamentary report on the subject. The report made 54 recommendations for social and legal

reforms.[1] Research was carried out in two stages between 1982 and 1986.

Stage 1 investigated the extent, nature and causes of domestic violence. Three major questionnaire surveys were conducted: a rural survey covering 19 villages in 16 provinces; a survey of the urban poor in Port Moresby; and a postal survey of urban elites. A total of 1,191 men and 1,203 women were interviewed in these surveys. Further data were provided by a survey of two squatter settlements in Port Moresby; a study of domestic violence victims seeking treatment at Lae's Angau Hospital; case studies of beaten wives; and three anthropological studies. The results have been published in four major volumes and numerous reports.[2]

Stage 2 examined existing remedies and their deficiencies, through analysis of:

- District and Local Court case files in five provinces
- A joint study with police on police records at three police stations in Port Moresby
- A study carried out in 15 provinces of police attitudes towards wife-beating
- Two anthropological studies of village courts
- Interviews with staff in the justice, health education and social service sectors, and dozens of discussions held as part of training sessions and workshops conducted by the LRC around the country
- Documents gathered from 38 countries and several international organisations describing strategies being tried elsewhere.

The LRC's research also investigated the frequency, duration and severity of domestic violence in the survey populations, the use of weapons, community responses, and other aspects.

Nature of domestic violence

The Law Reform Commission (LRC) found that many wives were hit or punched, hit with sticks, weapons, belts and belt buckles, kicked, pushed down, slammed against walls, burnt with fire or cigarettes, scalded by hot food or water, and even bitten. During the 1986 consultations, participants mentioned that guns were much more easily available than four years earlier, especially in the Highlands, and that sometimes guns were used to threaten or injure wives.

Most of the cases recorded in the provincial hospitals that were reviewed by the LRC involved broken bones, head injuries, organ damage and severe lacerations through being slashed with bush knives. Some of the cases were fatal, being listed as dead on arrival (DOA) in the register. Among the urban poor, the LRC found that one in six low-income women interviewed (not just those who had admitted to being beaten) needed hospital treatment for injuries caused by their husbands.[3] Other common injuries are deafness and brain damage from blows to the head. Psychological effects of such traumas can be long lasting, but they are not recorded in the data.

Domestic violence against wives often involves forced sex (marital rape). Half the married women interviewed said they had been forced into sex by their husbands, either by beating or by threats. Forced sex within marriage is legally defined as rape. It has serious consequences for women's reproductive health and is also a major factor in the spread of HIV/AIDS.

Physical abuse of wives is very often accompanied by emotional, social and economic abuse. Some women say that constant verbal abuse, insults and shaming by their husbands are harder to tolerate than the beatings. Emotional abuse erodes their self-confidence and makes women feel helpless and hopeless. This mental state makes it difficult for wives to help themselves, and also makes it frustrating for others trying to help them. Physically abusive husbands also often try to isolate their wives, cutting them off from family and friends and sometimes locking them up for hours or days. Frequently women are deprived of money, including their own earnings.

Extent of domestic violence

The LRC research found that on average, two-thirds of wives have been hit by their husbands. The inci-

Table 1: Incidence of domestic violence in PNG[4]

	Rural	Urban low-income	Urban elite
Husbands hitting wives:			
Wives who have been hit	67%	56%	62%
Husbands who have hit	66%	55%	62%
Wives hitting husbands:			
Husbands who have been hit	30%	37%	50%
Wives who have hit	33%	24%	49%

Table 2: Indicators of the relative seriousness of wife- and husband-beating[5]

	Females	Males
Patients seeking treatment for domestic violence injuries	97%	3%
Domestic violence victims seeking police assistance	94%	6%

dence is slightly lower among urban populations, however the frequency and severity of violence is greater in the urban environment. There is considerable variation across the country, with figures of close to 100% in some of the Highlands villages surveyed, and half that level in the Oro and New Ireland villages.

To avoid potential allegations of bias, the questionnaires asked men and women the same questions about their behaviours, beliefs and attitudes. Interviews were conducted in private. Responses from men and women showed almost perfect agreement about the extent of wife-beating, and very close agreement about the extent of wives hitting husbands. Table 1 indicates the percentage of victims and offenders who admitted incidences of husbands hitting their wives and wives striking their husbands.

Some wives do hit their husbands, but the usual motive for this is self-defence. Husbands and wives are not usually equal antagonists: husbands have greater physical strength, and social and economic power; wives are usually dependent on their husbands and risk losing everything if they defend themselves too vigorously. The relative seriousness of male versus female use of violence is suggested by the police and hospital data (presented in Table 2). Consequently, the LRC made wife-beating the main target of its recommendations, although all the proposed remedies would also be available to any beaten husbands.

Causes of domestic violence

The causes of domestic violence may be viewed on two levels. On the first (surface) level is the "perceived cause," or the incident that triggers a specific act of violence. The second level is that of underlying causes that relate to the overall social situation.

At the level of perceived causes, respondents to the LRC surveys suggested that in rural areas, sexual jealousy, a wife's failure to fulfil all her duties, and dislike of the spouse were the three main causes of problems in marriage leading to violence. Sexual jealousy includes a common situation where it is the husband who commits adultery, yet it is the wife who gets beaten because she complains or questions him about it.[6] A wife's "failure to fulfil all her duties" covers situations where the woman does

not cooperate sexually with her husband and he uses force to get his way; this is stated by many people to be the main cause of wife-beating. Other situations in this category include a wife not carrying out household tasks to her husband's satisfaction. Dislike of the spouse apparently relates to arranged marriages, still a common practice in rural areas.

In urban areas, the main perceived causes were alcohol abuse, sexual jealousy and money problems. Of course, alcohol itself is not a cause of violence but a contributing factor. Other factors that did not figure highly in the LRC's findings during the early 1980s, yet surfaced in the consultations held for the preparation of LRC's Parliamentary report, were gambling by women (particularly on poker machines) and drug use by men. Use of marijuana is a growing problem in urban areas and throughout the Highlands; the high potency of locally grown plants is anecdotally reported to be associated with violence and psychological disturbances.[7]

To discuss underlying causes is to recognise the widespread acceptance of domestic violence, particularly wife beating, as a part of normal life. There is a common attitude that the payment of bride price entitles a man to control his wife and to discipline her forcefully if he thinks it necessary. Table 3 shows LRC findings on attitudes to domestic violence. The majority of women as well as men in rural areas accept the use of violence by husbands. Interestingly, most rural men feel that it is "all right" for their wives to hit them. While urban acceptance of spousal hitting is lower than in rural areas, the findings indicate that a relatively high proportion of people see violence as a socially tolerated means of settling marital conflict. These data suggest the need for programmes to change attitudes and promote communication and management skills.

Furthermore, although violence is condoned by a high percentage of both males and females, the gender differences of opinion cannot be ignored. These differences reflect the unequal situation of men and women generally in PNG society and particularly within marriage. Reducing these inequalities in the country's cultural, social economic and political systems must therefore also form part of a long-term strategy to reduce domestic violence.

Other underlying causes of domestic violence identified by the LRC include:

- Stress caused by rapid socio-economic change
- Lack of communication between husbands and wives, leading to suspicion and distrust

and

- High background level of violence and aggression in many of the traditional cultures, which is being reinforced in modern circumstances by violent media, tribal fighting and civil war.

Table 3: Attitudes towards domestic violence[8]

	Males Agreeing	Females Agreeing
Is it all right for husbands to hit wives?		
Rural	67%	57%
Urban low-income	42%	25%
Urban elite	41%	36%
Is it all right for wives to hit husbands?		
Rural	53%	45%
Urban Low income	44%	33%
Urban elite	39%	37%

An aspect of "stress caused by rapid socio-economic change" that came out very strongly during the consultations held by the LRC in 1992 was the great increase in poverty. To give a single illustration, when the LRC was conducting its research, PNG's monetary unit, the *kina*, was worth US$1.25. By November 2001 the value of the *kina* had sunk to US$0.25 – losing four-fifths of its purchasing power in just over a decade. Since wages only marginally increased, the devaluation of the *kina* had a devastatingly negative impact on living standards, especially in urban areas. Rural people also need money for daily survival, but money is in short supply, causing great hardships. Money is needed for school fees, clothing, transport, kerosene, soap and other basic household items. Since the World Bank/ International Monetary Fund Structural Adjustment Programme began in 1995, people have had to pay for medical treatment in towns. Poverty pushes people past the limits of their patience. The effects of this are seen in the climbing crime rate (and the flourishing security industry), the high level of violence against the most vulnerable people, and the rising numbers of women and girls turning to commercial sex work for a living.

This is not to suggest that domestic violence occurs only among the poor. The LRC research found that domestic violence is common at all levels of society. However, the report highlights the need for a strong government focus on poverty alleviation.

A personal experience

In Papua New Guinea, violence against women has existed for as many years as I can remember. It is regarded as a "family affair" or a "marital affair": when a man acts violently against his wife or child, very little help is offered from outside the family – even by the law enforcers including the policemen on duty. The situation is markedly worse in traditional rural societies where women are more likely to be regarded as second-class citizens and the property of the men they marry.

It is common in my village for men to severely beat their wives when something goes wrong in the family; even if a child makes a mistake, the mother always gets the blame. Out of 20 men, only four or five would never beat their wives. These men either have aggressive or domineering wives or have a "don't care" attitude. As a result, non-violent men are not held up as examples for others to follow; instead they are considered effeminate. Yet there are men in PNG who genuinely respect their wives and are opposed to physically mistreating women. In fact, in PNG there is a small organisation still in its infancy called "Men Against Violence."

There was an incident that I personally witnessed and wish to relate as an example of domestic violence; similar beatings happened to many other women. Names are withheld for privacy's sake.

> A small woman was married to a husky, well-built man. She would be beaten for very minor things, such as not having food ready when her husband came home or not arriving on time at a feast with food. When one of their children broke a glass, lost a knife or tangled up fishing lines, the husband beat the children's mother.
>
> One of many incidents led to a lifetime of remorse for the husband who regularly beat his wife. Many years ago, around December 1983, the wife in this story returned from another town to her village. She had been gone for at least six months; relatives had taken her away to have medical treatment because she had been very ill. Initially, her husband went with her and stayed for some months, but returned to his village following an argument with his brother-in-law. In December when the brother of the husband took his annual recreational leave with his family, he took the woman home. It was a stormy day, so the boat that brought the family over did not go straight to the village; it offloaded its passengers on the other side of the island, so they had to walk a long distance to get to the village.
>
> When they arrived, the husband arranged a welcome feast for his brother and his family. The poor woman who had been sick a year before leaving the village had lost almost all her garden crops; neither of her husband's two other wives cared for her vegetable plot during her absence. As a result, she had no food available in the garden for

the feast. As the feast progressed, more people came and the husband eventually got hungry. So sometime during the course of the feast, he asked for some food from his first wife. The woman replied: "I have just returned from the mainland and I don't have any food to cook for you. Why don't you ask your other wives who have been here all the time?"

This was a reasonable reply, but to her husband it was an offence, an "unutterable" crime that deserved punishment. He got up and chased after the wife. Grabbing a big stick, he smashed it on her head. She fell down naked as she only had a piece of material wrapped around her, the typical attire of PNG village women. The husband then grasped hold of her hair that was so soft and thin that it broke in his hands. I tried to come to her rescue and protect her; he didn't stop but beat both of us. The man's brother came and attempted to restrain him, but the husband was so furious and powerful that he overcame all of us. As we were staggering, the eldest of the man's three sisters came and tried to stop him, but he continued to angrily strike us.

The man's adopted son (his sister's illegitimate son) was in a nearby house, heard the commotion, and ran out. He came upon the scene and realised what was happening. He had his own grudges: while the first wife had been away, the other two women did not treat him well. The son was so angry that he threw punches at his father. But this man was from the chief's family and nobody ever threw punches at him. He got so furious that he turned on his adopted son and tried to kill him with the big stick that he was holding. But the man's brother came between them, took hold of the stick and pulled it away from him.

The man cursed his son on the spot and sent him away to his natural father. He said to his son, "You illegitimate ingrate (editor's words) child. I took you under my care and brought you up to be a man and now you dare to punch at me. I promise you I will still be alive an old man and you will die before me."

Cultural factors

Culture plays a major role in the mistreatment of women and girls. In the PNG context women and girls are regarded as inferior, and are accorded second priority in inheritance. Men folk in a family still charge large amounts of money and wealth in bride price for their sisters and daughters. A young daughter in a remote mountain village has no say over whom she wants to marry. If an old man who is wealthy asks for a 14-, 15- or 16-year-old girl, the parents have no hesitation in agreeing if the man is willing to pay the bride price. As soon as the girl has her first menstruation, she will be given away to the man.

One such incident, which happened in one of World Vision Papua New Guinea's very remote project areas, caused great suffering not only to the female but also to the male involved:

> A sponsored child was attending the local primary school. While she was in school, her parents received money from a man much older than the girl and who was already married. The girl was about 15 or 16 years old and had a boyfriend at school. When her parents discovered that she had a boyfriend, they forbade her to see him, but she was so in love that she often sneaked off to meet him. One day she got caught and her father belted her very hard. The boy's older brother was also angry when he heard about the forbidden courtship; so angry that he threatened to kill his brother with an axe because the younger brother had brought shame to the family.
>
> The girl was so heartbroken that she ran away from the house. For a day and a night she was not to be found. Then after a search of the area she was discovered hanging by her neck from a tree in the forest. When her boyfriend heard about her suicide, he felt he couldn't live anymore. He went and demanded that his angry brother chop him to death with an axe while he stretched himself on the ground. The older brother took his axe and would have killed the younger brother if his wife had not pushed him away. The young man then got up, said to his brother: "Well if you don't want to kill me then I will kill myself." He got a rope, went into the bush and hung himself.

This is one story, but there are so many similar incidents. Likewise, sexual harassment and rape are prevalent social "diseases" in PNG. Some of the family and sexual violence in the country has been well researched and much is known about it. But there are numerous other cases that have not been researched and documented.

Raising awareness about rape

Rape and sexual assault are forms of violence against women and girls that extensive research has found to be very prevalent in PNG. For example, the LTS report contains citations of research done by the PNG Medical Research Institute in 1993. Researchers interviewed 423 men and women, and conducted 61 focus group discussions from cultural regions representing 82% of PNG's population. The study covered a wide range of aspects of sexual behaviour. One finding of the research was that "sexual violence is a major issue in the lives of men and women, with serious health consequences for the health of the PNG population."[9]

On 25 November 2001, PNG officially launched the International Day Against Violence Against Women. The Day, a Sunday, was observed with an ecumenical service organised by the National Women's Council and the PNG Council of Churches, and all churches were asked to observe the Day in their own services. (In PNG, it is normal for significant occasions to be celebrated beginning with a church service or prayer by a clergyman.) Main celebrations were held on Monday 26 November at a stadium in Port Moresby.

More recently, the National Council of Women and women's advocates conducted forums to raise public awareness on problems related to sexual violence. In 2001, for example, the Council called attention to rape. Concurrently, reports stated that family and sexual violence is increasing in PNG. Coping with these problems places a huge drain on the nation's already-overburdened health, police, courts, prison and probation, and welfare services.

Furthermore, family and sexual violence has serious consequences for individuals, families, communities and the nation as a whole. The scale of the problem is so great that no one is unaffected by its consequences. A report on the issue was completed in late 2001 and launched by Lady Roslyn Morauta, the wife of the Prime Minister, the Right Honourable Sir Mekere Morauta. Research was funded again by the British High Commissioner, Mr Simon Scadden. The British Government spent K126,000 on the report, and also provided financial assistance for the costs of workshops on family violence held since it was published.

While reaffirming the British Government's continued support, Mr. Scadden commented:

> "There is a conspiracy of silence that needs to be broken. Women and men throughout Papua New Guinea are beginning to speak out and assert their right to be heard."

Cases of rape were once rarely reported because they were not considered to be topics for public discussion. However, some brutal rapes and killings have changed that. One case involved an airline bus that was picking up female shift workers early in the morning. The bus was held up by gangsters, and three of the women in the vehicle were raped. The women were taken to Australia for counselling. Another example happened some years back in the urban town of Mount Hagen. A bus full of night shift nurses from the provincial hospital was hijacked and taken to an isolated place where all the women were raped. In partial response, all the nurses went on strike demanding more protection and assurance of safety from the government and the public.

In response to these tragic crimes, women's advocacy groups and concerned institutions have created awareness to the extent that rape has become a topic of concern and is no longer taboo. There were plans for a 16-day observance period during which the media will promote awareness of the theme of the day: "PNG Says No to Rape."

Closing

Violence against women is a tremendous problem in Papua New Guinea that requires a great deal of public education if it is to be addressed in a meaningful way. Awareness raising should also concentrate on educating women and girls on their rights

as human beings – that they have human and constitutional rights equal to those of men. Above all, women should be respected as created in God's own image. Men and boys need to understand that women were created by God to be helpmates and not objects of subjugation.

The church in Papua New Guinea needs to rise above cultural boundaries to engage in practical applications of the Word of God in dealing with issues such as the low status of women. Many church congregations need to take a hard look at themselves; there are churches in PNG that do not permit women to take an active role in the church, such as serving on church committees or sharing the Word of God from the pulpit. In this regard World Vision Papua New Guinea can have a role in raising awareness and facilitating understanding of the value of women as created beings made in the image and likeness of God.

References

1 Law Reform Commission (LRC), *Interim Report on Domestic Violence*, presented to Parliament on 3 March 1987, Port Moresby, 1992

2 Sources include: Bradley, C., "Wife beating in Papua New Guinea – Is it a Problem?" *Papua New Guinea Medical Journal*, Vol. 31, No. 4, 1988, pp. 257-268; Bradley, C., "Should Human Rights Apply to Wives? Wife-beating and the Work of the Papua New Guinea Law Reform Commission," *Legal Service Bulletin*, Monash University, Vol. 15, No. 5, 1990, pp. 18-21; Bradley, C., "Violence in Marriage in Urban Papua New Guinea: The Role of the Churches," *Catalyst. Journal of the Melanesian Institute*, Vol. 20, No. 2, 1990, pp. 137-156; and Toft, S. ed., "Domestic Violence in Papua New Guinea," Law Reform Commission Monograph No. 3, 1985, Boroko, PNG (anthropological studies of aspects of domestic violence in Papua New Guinea).

3 LRC, 1992, p. 17

4 LRC, 1992, pp. 16–17

5 LRC, 1992, p. 18

6 LRC, 1992, p. 21

7 Cox, E. *Campaigning Against Domestic Violence: An Evaluation of the Women and Law Committee's Campaign Against Domestic Violence 1986-1992*, Government of Papua New Guinea and UNICEF, September 1999, pp. 92–3

8 LRC, 1992, pp. 19–20

9 National Sex and Reproduction Research Team and Carol Jenkins, *National Study of Sexual and Reproductive Behaviour in Papua New Guinea*, Monograph No. 10, Goroka: PNG Institute of Medical Research, 1994

World Vision is a Christian relief and development partnership which serves more than 85 million people in some 80 countries. World Vision seeks to follow Christ's example by working with the poor and oppressed in the pursuit of justice and human transformation.

Children are often most vulnerable to the effects of poverty. World Vision works with each partner community to ensure that children are able to enjoy improved nutrition, health and education. Where children live in especially difficult circumstances, surviving on the streets, suffering in exploitative labour, or exposed to the abuse and trauma of conflict, World Vision works to restore hope and to bring justice.

World Vision recognises that poverty is not inevitable. Our Mission Statement calls us to challenge those unjust structures, which constrain the poor in a world of false priorities, gross inequalities and distorted values. World Vision desires that all people are able to reach their God-given potential, and thus works for a world which no longer tolerates poverty.

Violence Against Women:

From Silence to ***Empowerment***

World Vision House
599 Avebury Boulevard
Central Milton Keynes
Bucks, MK9 3PG
England

World Vision Advocacy Office
222 East 48th Street
New York, NY 10017

International Liaison Office
6, Chemin de la Tourelle
Geneva, CH 1209
Switzerland

EU Liaison Office
22 Rue de Toulouse
B-1040 Brussels
Belgium

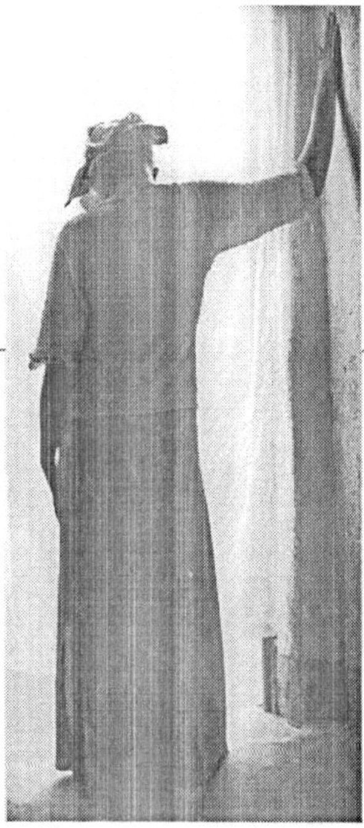

www.globalsociety.org
www.developmentstudies.org

World Vision

World Vision Publications
800 West Chestnut Ave
Monrovia, CA 91016-3198 USA
www.wvi.org
www.worldvision.org

ISBN 1-887983-54-6

9 781887 983549